NOW THERE'S AN EASY WAY TO CUT DOWN ON FATS.

Over a million and a half readers of *The All-in-One Calorie Counter* and *The All-in-One Carbohydrate Gram Counter* can attest to the advantages of having such a valuable source at their fingertips. Now, well-known nutrition expert Jean Carper has created another convenient and important handbook—*The All-in-One Low Fat Gram Counter*. The fat content in over 4,000 foods—both fresh and processed—is listed in easy-to-find, alphabetical order. Every entry is based on the most up-to-date information available from food manufacturers and the U. S. Department of Agriculture.

AN INVALUABLE BOOK IF YOU ARE CONCERNED ABOUT YOUR HEALTH.

Bantam Books by Jean Carper
Ask your bookseller for the books you have missed

THE ALL-IN-ONE CALORIE COUNTER
THE ALL-IN-ONE CARBOHYDRATE GRAM COUNTER
THE ALL-IN-ONE LOW FAT GRAM COUNTER
THE BRAND NAME NUTRITION COUNTER

The All-In-One Low Fat Gram Counter

By Jean Carper

BANTAM BOOKS · TORONTO · NEW YORK · LONDON

🚩

THE ALL-IN-ONE LOW FAT GRAM COUNTER
A Bantam Book / June 1980

ISBN 0–553–13982–7

Published simultaneously in the United States and Canada

Bantam Books are published by Bantam Books, Inc. Its trade-
mark, consisting of the words "Bantam Books" and the por-
trayal of a bantam, is Registered in U.S. Patent and Trademark
Office and in other countries. Marca Registrada. Bantam
Books, Inc., 666 Fifth Avenue, New York, New York 10019.

PRINTED IN THE UNITED STATES OF AMERICA

0 9 8 7 6 5 4 3 2 1

Contents

Introduction	ix
How To Use This Book	xix
Abbreviations	xxxiv
Appetizers	1
Baby Food	3
Baking Powder	15
Beer, Ale, Malt Liquor	16
Biscuits	16
Bread	17
Butter and Margarine	21
Cakes	25
Candy	33
Cereals	36
Cheese	42
Chewing Gum	45
Chinese Foods	45
Chips, Crisps and Similar Snacks	47
Chocolate and Chips	49
Cocktail Mixes	50
Cocoa	50
Coconut	51
Coffee	51
Condiments	52
Cookies	53
Corn Starch	60
Crackers	60
Cream	62
Dessert Mixes	63
Diet Bars	63
Dinners	64
Eggs	71

Fish and Seafood 73
Flavoring, Sweet 80
Flour, Meal and Grains 80
Frostings 82
Fruit 84
Fruits and Fruit Juices and Drinks 85
Gelatin 87
Gravies 87
Health Foods 91
Herbs and Spices 92
Ice Cream and Similar Frozen Products 93
Italian Foods 96
Jams, Jellies, Preserves, Butters, Marmalade 99
Liqueurs and Brandies 101
Macaroni 103
Mayonnaise 104
Meat 105
Mexican Foods 119
Milk 121
Muffins: English and Sweet 123
Noodles and Noodle Dishes 127
Nuts 128
Oils 133
Olives 133
Pancakes, Waffles and Similar Breakfast Foods 135
Pastry 137
Pickles and Relishes 139
Pies 140
Pizza 145
Popcorn 147
Pot Pies 148
Poultry and Poultry Entrees 149
Pretzels 153
Pudding 154
Rice and Rice Dishes 159
Rolls and Buns 161
Salad Dressings 165
Sauces 169
Seasoning Mixes 172
Shortening 174

Soft Drinks 174
Soups 175
Spaghetti and Spaghetti Dishes 188
Spreads 189
Sugar and Sweeteners 191
Tea 193
Toppings 193
Vegetables 195
Vegetable Juices 217
Wines 219
Yeast 221
Yogurt 221

Fast Foods 225

Index 235

The Case Against Fat

You're a rare individual if you're not eating too much fat. And it is not good for you. Many people report they simply feel better, more vigorous and energetic when they cut down on fatty foods. There's also sound scientific evidence that if you eat less fat you're less likely to suffer from overweight and such chronic diseases as high blood pressure, heart disease, and cancer.

Many people do want to change their diets and eliminate many fatty foods but have only a scant idea of which foods are highest in fat. That's the purpose of this book: to give you a complete guide to the fat content of both fresh and processed foods.

HOW MUCH YOU SHOULD CUT DOWN

Americans on the average now eat over 40 percent of their calories daily in fat. That's not extraordinary when compared with European or Scandanavian countries, where dairy products are common. All so-called Western diets are high in fat. In comparison, many Oriental and African diets where grain is the main staple, instead of meats and dairy products, are low in fats. The pre-World War II Japanese, subsisting on rice and fish, ate about 10 percent of their calories in fat. But with the influence of the Western world, the Japanese diet has been changing and going up in fat. So, too, has the incidence of Western-type diseases, mainly heart disease and cancer.

The consumption of fat in the U.S. has been rising since the turn of the century. The number of calories we consume daily has barely changed since 1910, nor has the proportion of calories that come from protein. But, the amount of those calories that come from *fat* has gone up

25 percent. And the number of calories attributed to carbohydrates (except sugar) has dropped by an equal percentage. In other words, we have almost directly replaced our complex carbohydrates, notably grains, with fat.

You're eating on the average about 2½ tablespoons more fat today than an American at the turn of the century—or 24 pounds more fat a year. Most of that rise is attributed to salad and cooking oils; however, recently meat, namely beef, has become the primary contributor to the rise in fat intake.

Health specialists almost unanimously agree that most people are eating too much fat. Some say we should not eat more than one third or 30 percent of our calories in fat. For example, Senator George McGovern's nutrition subcommittee in its well-publicized "dietary goals" recommended reducing the fat intake to one third of calories and replacing it with grains, fruits, and vegetables.

Others, like Nathan Pritikin, founder of the famed Pritikin diet, which has had remarkable results for some people, believe the fat reduction should be much more severe. Pritikin favors eating only 5 to 10 percent of your calories in fat, which means a massive change to an exceedingly low-fat diet and the exclusion of certain high-fat foods.

Pritikin and an increasing number of other health experts are recommending cutting down on all kinds of fat—saturated, or animal, fats as well as unsaturated, or vegetable, fats. They believe that excessive amounts of either or both are dangerous to your health.

FAT AND HEART DISEASE

A high-fat diet can contribute to heart disease in two ways—directly and indirectly. One way is by putting saturated fats into the body, which raises the blood cholesterol believed to lead to atherosclerosis and heart disease. And the second way is by replacing the complex carbohydrates in the diet that may lower cholesterol, protecting against heart disease. Studies show that when people cut down on fat in the diet, they automatically eat more carbohydrates, such as whole grains and vegetables.

Countless studies have been done both on animals and humans showing that high blood cholesterol levels are related to heart disease and that the cholesterol can be lowered through a low saturated fat, low cholesterol diet. At least fifteen expert committees on dietary fat and heart disease have recommended lowering the intake of the percentage of calories derived from fat to between 25 and 35 percent. After a comprehensive study of the literature on diet and heart disease, Dr. Jeremiah Stamler, writing in the medical journal *Circulation*, July 1978, concluded: "It is reasonable and sound to designate 'rich' (high-fat) diet as a primary, essential, necessary cause of the current epidemic of premature atherosclerotic disease raging in the western industrialized countries."

Generally cholesterol is blamed as the main culprit. Thus, some people will cut down on high cholesterol foods such as shrimp and eggs and still go on eating high-fat foods such as beef and coconut. What they don't realize is that these saturated, high-fat foods also raise cholesterol levels in the blood—even more so than high-cholesterol foods do. Patricia Hausman, a nutritionist at the Center for Science in the Public Interest, a Washington D.C. based public interest group specializing in health and nutrition, points out that just because foods are low in cholesterol does not necessarily mean they are all right for your arteries.

Yet, meat and dairy producers sometimes tout their products as low in cholesterol, never mentioning they are high in fat. Here is a quote from a flyer from the National Livestock and Meat Board: "Steaks, chops and roasts are not full of cholesterol as many have come to believe. . . . Many people are adjusting their diets to control cholesterol by eating less meat and butter, fewer eggs and more poultry and fish. Yet, according to the Meat Board, meat is lower in cholesterol than a number of poultry, fish and seafood items."

The Dairy Council publicizes that milk and other dairy products are not high in cholesterol. And the candy bar makers will tell you that chocolate is not high in cholesterol. It is true, of course, but it can be misleading. For although meat, milk, cheese, and chocolate may not be high in cholesterol, they are high in saturated fats that can raise cholesterol levels in the blood.

Ms. Hausman writes: "Talking only about the cholesterol in foods and not mentioning saturated fat is a common tactic of the meat and dairy industries. The public associates cholesterol in food with cholesterol in the blood, well aware that the higher their blood cholesterol levels, the greater the risk of heart disease and in some cases, stroke. But fewer people know that saturated fat also increases their blood cholesterol—even more so than the cholesterol in foods. The dairy and meat industries try to hide this fact because high-fat dairy products and many meats have a hefty share of saturated fat."

Hausman says that although shrimp is exceptionally high in cholesterol, it actually raises the cholesterol in your blood to about the same extent as a piece of lean meat that has only moderate amounts of cholesterol. The high fat content of the meat does the trick.

Thus, if you want to cut down on true blood cholesterol levels, you must also curtail your intake of highly saturated fats.

Further, replacing fatty foods with carbohydrates may have a protective effect against heart disease. Studies show that those with a low incidence of coronary heart disease —mainly vegetarians—consume from 65 to 85 percent of their diet in carbohydrates from whole grains (mainly cereals) and vegetables (mainly potatoes). Dr. Stamler also points out that Southern Italians, who have a starchy diet (about 40 to 55 percent of their calories from carbohydrates), have lower blood cholesterol levels.

Although heart specialists for years have condemned saturated fats, there is increasing evidence that unsaturated fats too may be more detrimental than previously believed. Pritikin claims that "all excess fats are bad for you, animal and vegetable, saturated and unsaturated." For one reason, he says, because fats of all kinds have a suffocating effect on the blood. He says eating too much fat encloses part of the blood in a fatty film, causing clumps to form that plug up small blood vessels, resulting in a shut down of from 5 to 20 percent of your blood circulation. He also says unsaturated fats such as vegetable oils can boost the levels of triglycerides—fatty acids also linked to heart disease.

Although the conventional wisdom in recent years has been to substitute unsaturated fats, such as margarine, for saturated fats, such as butter, to prevent heart disease, some new questions are being raised about the safety of margarine. Some studies suggest that when margarine is hydrogenated (hardened) it forms new molecular structures that could be detrimental to the body. Dr. Hugh Sinclair, at the Laboratory of Human Nutrition at Oxford University in England, found that hydrogenated fats caused a deficiency of essential fatty acids in the bodies of both animals and humans. He said such a deficiency "contributed to neurological diseases, heart disease, arteriosclerosis, skin disease, various degenerative conditions such as cataract and arthritis and cancer."

At the University of Illinois, food chemistry professor Fred Kummerow fed pigs hydrogenated fat containing high amounts of trans fatty acids and found that 58 percent of them developed early signs of atherosclerosis. That was compared with only 14 percent for those not fed the hydrogenated fat. Interestingly, the animals fed the hydrogenated fat had higher levels of cholesterol in the blood.

Recently, a scientist in Israel, Professor S. Hillel Blondheim, found evidence, after a two-year study, contradicting the traditional views of heart disease and diet. He found that a group of Bedouin who had become Westernized and ate more unsaturated fats had a higher level of blood cholesterol than tribesmen who ate saturated fats. Said Professor Blondheim: "Here's a population among whom incidence of heart disease was nil, although all the fat in the traditional diet was of animal origin. Now those in steady contact with westernized culture appear to be consuming more polyunsaturates; and yet, as far as we can tell from the limited number of cases in our sample, they are precisely the ones who have higher levels of serum cholesterol. This might knock the accepted theories into a cocked hat."

Obviously, not everything is known about the effects of fats of all kinds on heart disease, but there is sufficient evidence to show that it is detrimental and that perhaps the safest course of all, as some scientists recommend, is to cut down on the consumption of all kinds of fat—saturated and unsaturated, animal and vegetable.

FAT AND CANCER

There's also increasing evidence that fats of all kinds, both animal and vegetable, may be related to cancer. The evidence is not conclusive, but it is compelling enough that the National Cancer Institute recently recommended reducing the fat content in the diet to one third of the calories as a possible way of preventing cancer.

The theory has been promoted vigorously by Dr. Ernst Wynder, head of the American Health Foundation and a prominent cancer researcher. Dr. Wynder in 1965 presented a paper showing a worldwide correlation between eating high amounts of animal fat and high rates of colon cancer. He said this pattern, tieing colon cancer to the "high-fat Western diet," was clear in this country, the Netherlands, Belgium, Denmark, West Germany, France, England, and Canada. In contrast, he noted that the Japanese, who at the time ate one fourth as much animal fat as we do, had a colon cancer rate of only 2.5 per 100,000 compared with 14 per 100,000 in the United States.

Further, the Japanese who move to this country develop higher rates of cancer. The reasonable explanation, says Dr. Wynder, is a change in the diet. Also, animal studies dating back to the 1930s and 1940s show that animals exposed to cancer-causing chemicals develop more cancers when they are fed high fat diets.

The theory lately has gathered more advocates. And a high-fat diet has now been linked by many studies to several kinds of cancer: notably breast, but also cancer of the prostate, pancreas, ovaries, kidney, and bladder.

At first Dr. Wynder and others believed that cancer was associated only with animal, or saturated, fats. But lately that theory has been turned topsy-turvy. Recent, well-respected tests show that vegetable, or unsaturated, fats may be even a more potent cancer producer than animal fats. Kenneth Carroll, a biochemist at the University of Ontario, showed that when you feed carcinogen-exposed rats high amounts of unsaturated fats—such as olive, corn, and safflower oil—they develop twice as many tumors as rats exclusively fed saturated fats such as butter and meat fat.

What's more, when you mix only small amounts of unsaturated fats (3 percent of the diet) with saturated fats, you get even more cancer in rats than you would with either alone. The unsaturated fats somehow potentiate the cancer production.

Nobody at this point knows why this happens, but Carroll and other experts, in the absence of more precise knowledge, advise that everyone should severely reduce their fat intake—of all kinds—as a precaution against cancer. At the moment, many cancer scientists are advising cutting back to at least 30 percent of calories from fat—the same amount generally recommended by heart specialists. However, this may not be enough to prevent cancer.

Dr. John Weisburger, a well-known cancer researcher working at the American Health Foundation with Dr. Wynder, points out we may have to reduce our fat intake even further—perhaps to 20 or even 10 percent of calories. He notes that prior to World War II, the Japanese, when they had an exceptionally low rate of cancer, were eating only 10 percent of their calories in fat. This is along the lines recommended by the Pritikin diet. Dr. Weisburger notes that studies on animals in England have shown that animals who ate 30 percent of their calories in fat had just as high a rate of cancer as those who ate 60 percent of their calories in fat. So, he suggests, the cutback to 30 percent may not be severe enough to prevent cancer; more studies, he says, are needed to define more precisely the permissible amount of fat.

However, there's another avenue of benefit. At the same time you reduce your fat content, you will eat more vegetables and grain, and they in themselves may protect you from cancer. There is evidence that a higher consumption of grains and fruits and vegetables will reduce the chances of cancer. One theory is that fiber in grain (cereals and whole-grain breads) protects against cancer; thus, the National Cancer Institute also recommends increasing fiber as you cut fat. Another theory is that the vegetables themselves contain specific chemicals that counteract the effects of cancer. This is not as off-the-wall as it may sound at first.

Dr. Saxon Graham, at the State University of New York at Buffalo, found that people who ate the most cabbage—yes, plain old cabbage, whether cooked or raw, as sauerkraut or cole slaw—were less likely to have colon cancer. Further, a chemical has been isolated from such vegetables that does prevent cancer in laboratory animals. Professor Lee Wattenberg at the University of Minnesota found that a chemical called "indoles" reduces the rate of cancer in animals exposed to cancer-causing substances. Dr. Wattenberg exposed animals to carcinogenic substances and at the same time gave some of them indoles. In one test 81 percent of the rats who did *not* get indoles developed breast cancer. But only 21 to 27 percent of the rats given indoles as an antidote developed breast cancer.

The important point is that these indoles are found naturally in certain vegetables, including cabbage. Other vegetables that also have indoles are brussels sprouts, turnips, cauliflower, and broccoli. Perhaps it's not surprising then that vegetarians often have a lower cancer rate than meat eaters.

How a high-fat diet might produce cancer is unknown. But scientists, including Dr. Wynder, believe fat is not a direct initiator of cancer (in the way pesticides are). Instead, they believe it is a "cancer promoter." In other words, eating fat somehow encourages the cancer to grow. It might do this, Wynder theorizes, by causing the body through complicated mechanisms to produce substances that promote cancer growth. For example, according to Dr. Wynder, excessive fat produces high amounts of bile acids in the colon, and bile acids have produced cancer in laboratory animals. Also, studies show that colon cancer victims often have higher concentrations of bile acids.

As for breast cancer, the theory is that a high-fat diet encourages a disproportionate production of a hormone called prolactin. Prolactin has been proved as a cancer promoter in animals. Further, Wynder has shown that women who go on low-fat vegetarian diets produce less prolactin than when they're eating high-fat meats.

Although all the evidence is not in, many believe it is sufficiently persuasive to encourage people to reduce their fat intake to prevent cancer. Dr. Wynder strongly believes that women who already have breast cancer should cut down on fatty foods to slow the growth of cancer. Even if the evidence is not firm, many scientists say cutting down on fat certainly can't hurt you, and it will do your general health and weight a lot of good.

FAT AND OTHER HEALTH PROBLEMS

One of the greatest dangers of overdosing on fatty foods is getting fat yourself. It is very difficult to continue day after day on a high-fat diet and control your weight. Studies show that people with severe weight problems usually consume high quantities of fatty foods.

Not only is overweight a problem in itself, it leads to other health problems. Dr. Theodore Cooper, former assistant secretary for health, has said: "Overweight aggravates cardiovascular disease and osteoarthritis, and increases the liability to hypertension, atherosclerosis, hernia and gallbladder disease. It may also facilitate the emergence of latent diabetes in predisposed individuals as they approach an advanced age and adds to the hazards of surgery. . . . Statistics make it quite clear that the obese do not live as long as the lean. The chief cause of death among overweight individuals is cardiovascular-renal diseases, diabetes and disorders of the liver and biliary tract (the gallbladder.)"

Additionally, fatty foods are often not very nutritious; and consuming them in place of better foods, such as grains and fruits and vegetables, deprives you of nutrients. Fats such as salad oils and lard provide relatively empty calories—little different in nutrient value from the calories from alcohol and sugar—that produce energy and weight gain but little else.

In fact, fat is the most fattening nutrient of all. One fat gram has 9 calories. That's compared with only 4 calories for one gram of carbohydrate or one gram of protein. Thus, a fat gram is more than twice as fattening as either a protein or carbohydrate gram—even a gram of pure sugar.

Small wonder then that for all kinds of reasons experts say you will be much healthier and feel better if you become aware of which foods are high in fat and restrict them in your diet. This book will help you do that.

How to Use This Book

WHAT THE FIGURES MEAN

This book gives the total number of fat grams (a combination of both saturated and unsaturated fat) per serving sizes. The "fat gram" is the scientific measurement used to express the fat content of a food. A gram is a measure of weight; there are 28.5 grams in one ounce. So, if an ounce of a certain food contains 14 grams of fat, about half of the food by weight is fat. If a cup of whole milk weighs 244 grams and has 8.5 grams of fat, it is 3.5 percent fat by weight.

However, because most of the milk is water, the percent of fat by weight does not provide the final judgment on how fat the food really is. Three percent seems low indeed. But whole milk is considered a *high-fat food*. The reason is that nearly 50 percent of its calories come from fat. Fat is one of three nutrients that supply calories; the other two nutrients are protein and carbohydrates. Thus, a food that derives a high percentage of its calories from protein is called a high-protein food; one that gets a large percentage of its calories from sugar or carbohydrate is a high-carbohydrate food. The same with fat.

The accepted way to judge whether a food is high or low fat is to note what percentage of its calories come from fat. This is a principle widely used by nutritional experts.

In this book, therefore, you will find a second column showing what percentage of the calories in a food come from fat. This will tell you at a glance whether the food falls into the category of high fat, moderate fat or low fat.

The percentages are listed in increments of ten, showing the range a food falls into. For example, 0–10 percent, 50–60 percent, 90–100 percent, and so on. Because the fat grams are often rounded off after calculation* and 9 calories per gram is an average (it can vary by decimal points), it is impossible to be absolutely precise on the percentages. What is important is that the percentages will instantly warn you of the high-fat content.

All the figures in this book came either from the company producing the food or, in the case of generic and fresh foods, from the U.S. Department of Agriculture.

HIDDEN FATS IN FOODS

Some foods are obviously high in fat—lard, butter, vegetable oils, the fat part of meats. But that is only a small part of the story. Most of the fat we eat is hidden—either in the tissues of lean means, such as steaks, or in processed foods, such as chocolate cakes. Many people don't realize that many of the high calorie foods are so fattening because of their high fat content. Further, some so-called "health foods," such as granola cereals, avocados, and sunflower seeds, are high-fat foods.

Here are some special foods to take note of if you're on a low-fat diet:

- **Coconut and palm oil.** Coconut meat is one of the highest fatty foods around, deriving about 85 percent of its calories from fat. The oil of both coconut and palm, widely used in processed foods, is 100 percent fat, like other cooking oils. However, coconut oil and palm oil, unlike other vegetable oils, are very highly saturated—even more highly saturated than beef fat. Coconut oil is *twice* as saturated as lard, and palm oil is just as saturated as beef tallow or butter. And the tragedy is that many people who give up whole milk and cream be-

---

*The precision with which food companies report their fat gram information varies.

cause of its saturated fat content use products made with coconut oil.

One woman, advised by her heart specialists to avoid cream and whole milk, started using one of the liquid nondairy creamers every morning on her cereal; its primary base was coconut oil. She undid in a short time all the good derived from restricting other saturated fats in her diet. Skim milk, which is very low in fat, would have been a solution. Check the labels of processed foods to see if they contain coconut or palm oil; most of the nondairy creamers and other nondairy products do.

- **Granola cereals.** Although cereals in general are low in fat, granola is an exception. It may have slightly more protein, calcium, riboflavin, and niacin than other cereals, but this benefit does not offset the drawback: five to six times as much fat per serving as other cereals. The fat usually comes from coconut. Though highly touted as a "health food," granola, when you're cutting down on fat, is not as good as a lower fat, high fiber cereal, such as plain bran or bran flakes.
- **Avocados.** On a low-fat diet, you can usually eat all the fruit you want. They are packed with nutrients and are low in calories. But avocados are a major exception. An avocado is very fatty, with over 80 percent of its calories from fat. Its fat is unsaturated, but avocado is definitely a food to avoid when you're on a low-fat diet.
- **Peanuts, peanut butter, and all kids of nuts.** Except for chestnuts they are all high in fat—in the 70 to 90 percent of calories range. Nuts are also very high in trace minerals, but you can also get those much-needed minerals from other sources, such as grains, without getting such a high dose of fat and calories.
- **Chocolate.** Chocolate is naturally high in fat (saturated), which is the main reason it tastes so rich. Milk chocolate gets over 50 percent of its calories from fat. Thus when you eat a chocolate candy bar, most of the calories come from the fat instead of the sugar. The same is true of some baked goods containing chocolate.
- **Red meats.** Ironically, the better grade of beef you buy,

the higher its fat content and of course its price. The federal government has structured the meat-grading system so that the more marbling (fat streaks) a steak has, the better grade it gets. Actually, lesser grades of beef are leaner than prime beef, but they're also tougher. Most American beef is fattened on grain, instead of grass, which accounts for its high fat content.

Most important, it's essential when cutting down on fat, to trim off as much fat as possible from red meats. However, that will only partly do the trick. Meat, even in its leanest portions is intrinsically high in fat. Well-trimmed beef rib roast and pork loin roast still derive about 50 percent of their calories from fat. Processed meats, such as luncheon meats and notably hot dogs, are very high in fat—getting around 80 percent of their calories from fat. Certainly hot dogs are not foods for people on low-fat diets.

On the other hand, chicken and turkey with the skin removed are relatively much lower in fat, especially white meat.

FOODS THAT ARE GOOD FOR YOU

• **Pasta** (spaghetti, noodles, macaroni). It's difficult to convince people—especially those who want to lose weight—that pasta is good for them. Starchy foods, having the reputation as peasant foods, are some of the best you can eat for your health—mainly because of their low fat content. Plain noodles and spaghetti get only 10 to 20 percent of their calories from fat; and if you top them with tomato sauce containing only a little oil and no cheese or meat, the combination is extremely low in fat and consequently calories. Even frozen and fast-food pizzas have less fat than other such fast-foods as hamburgers and french fries. Of course, if you drench pasta with cream sauces and cheese—such as in making fettucine alfredo—you end up with a high-fat dish. Otherwise, if you want a low-fat, nutritious food, check out pasta.

- **Bread.** The first thing so many people say when they're going on diets is "I'm going to cut out bread." Yet, bread is very low in fat (and thus calories) and whole grain bread is very nutritious. Also, there's evidence bread is a good diet food. Professor Olaf Mickelsen of Michigan State University reported in *Cereal Foods World:* "Contrary to what most people think, bread in large amounts is an ideal food in a weight-reducing regimen. Recent work in our laboratory indicates that slightly overweight young men lost weight in a painless and practically effortless manner when they included 12 slices of bread per day in their program. That bread was eaten with their meals." What happened, says Professor Mickelsen, is that the dieters became so full because of the bread's bulk that they couldn't eat their usual number of calories from other foods. Though the dieters, he says, at as much of most foods as they wanted (and cut out only very high-calorie foods), they lost an average of 12.7 pounds in eight weeks.

- **Vegetables.** Almost all plain vegetables are low in fat, and you could eat as many as possible without overdoing it or gaining weight. Even potatoes, much maligned, are a very low-calorie food with only trace amounts of fat. What you must watch out for is the way vegetables are cooked (fried) or doused with cream, cheese, and butter sauces. These raise their fat content astronomically. Be especially aware of low-fat frozen vegetables, such as broccoli and peas, that are creamed or served au gratin. Their fat content sometimes goes up ten times or more.

- **Buttermilk.** Because of its rich sounding name, some people believe buttermilk contains lots of butter and is therefore high in fat. It's not. Actually, buttermilk is what's left after the fat solids that go to make butter have been removed. The buttermilk you find in supermarkets usually has been thickened by a bacterial process somewhat the way yogurt is. That thickness, however, does not come from fat. Buttermilk generally has about one fourth as much fat as whole milk. And butter-

milk made from skim milk is much lower in fat—
having only one eighth the amount of fat as whole milk.
So it is a relatively low-fat diet food.

SOME HIGH-FAT FOODS
(Over 50 percent of calories from fat)

Bacon
Hot dogs
Cream cheese
Hard cheeses
Mayonnaise and salad dressings
Peanuts
Avocados
Coconut
Butter
Eggs
Whipping cream
Hamburger (regular)
Beef, pork, and lamb roasts with fat

SOME LOW-FAT FOODS
(Less than 20 percent of calories from fat)

Cereals (except granola)
Bread
Rice
Fruits (except avocados)
Vegetables (except soybeans)
Skim milk
Low-fat cottage cheese
Egg whites
Plain pasta, spaghetti, noodles, macaroni
Fresh fish and most shellfish

HOW MANY FAT GRAMS YOU SHOULD EAT

Number of Fat Grams Allowed Per Day on Various Diets

Calories per day	30% calories in fat	20% calories in fat	10% calories in fat
3000	100	66	33
2500	83	55	27
2000	66	44	22
1500	50	33	16
1000	33	22	11

This chart shows how much you must cut back in fat grams to restrict your fat intake. For example, if you're eating 2000 calories per day, you're most likely eating at least 89 grams of fat per day (40 percent of calories, nine calories in each fat gram). If you want to cut back to 30 percent of calories, you can eat only 66 fat grams per day; if you want only 20 percent of your calories in fat, you are allowed 44 fat grams per day. And at 10 percent of calories—only 22 fat grams daily.

Most Americans now are taking in between 2000 and 3000 calories per day.

HOW TO TELL SATURATED FROM UNSATURATED FATS

Doctors sometimes make a distinction between "saturated" and "unsaturated" fats. Technically this is a distinction in the chemical makeup of the fatty acids. Saturated fat has a hydrogen atom attached to each of its carbon atoms in the chain; unsaturated fat has at least two carbon atoms to which no hydrogen atom is attached. However, the fatty acids in foods are not entirely saturated or unsaturated. All kinds of foods—meats, dairy products, vegetables—have varying amounts of saturated and unsaturated fats. So a food is not *exclusively* a saturated or unsaturated fatty food. A food is said to be high in saturated fat when the fat content is predominately one or the other. For example, the fat in safflower oil is 74 percent unsaturated; thus it is referred to as an unsaturated, or often a polyunsaturated, fatty food. In contrast, butter and beef fat are around 50 percent saturated fat; thus, they are called saturated fatty foods.

You will not find the fat grams in this book broken down into percentages of saturated and unsaturated fats. The premise of this book, which is consistent with much current scientific and nutritional thinking, is that it is wise to cut down on fat per se—regardless of whether it is saturated or unsaturated.

However, if you are more concerned about saturated fats, all you need to know as a rule is that saturated fats are found primarily in animal foods—meat, eggs, milk, cream, cheese. And the fat in vegetable products is mostly unsaturated. Fish, too, is low in saturated fats. The dramatic exceptions to this rule are coconut and palm oil, both highly saturated in fat content.

CHOLESTEROL CONTENT OF FOODS

Cholesterol, though technically not a fat, is a chemical component of animal fats; it is a waxy fatlike substance that does not dissolve in water or blood. The theory is that excessive cholesterol in the blood clumps and attaches itself to artery walls, leading to formation of "arterial plaque." As plaque builds up, it closes off arteries and helps cause heart attacks and strokes in some persons. Heart experts believe that the amount of cholesterol in the blood (serum cholesterol) is strongly predictive of the chances of having a heart attack—at least up until age fifty. After that other factors may be more important.

An expert study group recently convened by the American Health Foundation reported that average blood cholesterol levels among Americans are alarmingly high, even among children, and that they should be reduced by 25 percent. Although many physicians tell patients their cholesterol count is "normal" if it's no higher than 250 milligrams of cholesterol per deciliter, the study group agreed that the average level should be no more than 180 to 190. Dr. Henry Blackburn, director of the Laboratory of Physiological Hygiene at the University of Minnesota, says 150 to 160 is "ideal" to prevent heart attacks and artery disease.

Cholesterol—like fat—is *not* found in vegetable products in any significant amount. However, you may have noticed that some food companies advertise "cholesterol free" peanut-butter, "cholesterol free" mayonnaise and even "cholesterol free" cereals. Technically this is correct, but it has no meaning. Such advertising campaigns are meant to exploit an unknowledgable public.

Remember:
- You don't have to worry about vegetable products having cholesterol, regardless of the brand. Only animal products have cholesterol.
- Even taking the fat off meats does not eliminate cholesterol. Cholesterol is found in the lean parts of meats as well as the fat.
- Shellfish and organ meats such as liver, kidney, and brains, and egg yolks are particularly high in cholesterol.

Most Americans are now eating between 600 and 800 milligrams of cholesterol every day. Many experts think that should be cut to at least 300 milligrams per day. Pritikin says on his extremely low-fat diet, you only eat 100 milligrams of cholesterol per day.

By cutting down on animal and dairy fats, and eating more grains and vegetables—which do not have a smidgen of cholesterol and very little fat—you automatically reduce your intake of cholesterol radically.

Here is a list of the cholesterol content of some common foods:

Food	Amount	(Milligrams) Cholesterol
Milk, skim, fluid, or reconstituted dry	1 cup	5
Cottage cheese, uncreamed	½ cup	7
Mayonnaise, commercial	1 tbsp	10
Lard	1 tbsp	12
Yogurt, made from fluid and dry nonfat milk, plain or vanilla	carton (227 gm)	17
Cream, light table	1 fluid ounce	20

Food	Amount	(Milligrams) Cholesterol
Cottage cheese, creamed	½ cup	24
Cheese, pasteurized, processed American	28 gm (about 1 ounce)	25
Cheese, pasteurized, processed Swiss	28 gm (about 1 ounce)	26
Cream, half and half	¼ cup	26
Ice cream, regular, approximately 10% fat	½ cup	27
Cheese, cheddar	1 ounce	28
Milk, whole	1 cup	34
Sausage, frankfurter, all meat, cooked	1 frank	34
Butter	1 tbsp	35
Beef and vegetable stew, canned	1 cup	36
Cake, baked from mix, yellow 2 layer, made with eggs, water, chocolate frosting	75 gm	36
Oysters, salmon	3 ounces, cooked	40
Clams, halibut, tuna	3 ounces, cooked	55
Chicken, turkey, light meat	3 ounces, cooked	67
Beef, pork, lobster, chicken, turkey, dark meat	3 ounces, cooked	75
Lamb, veal, crab	3 ounces, cooked	85
Tuna, canned in oil, drained solids	184 gm	116
Lobster, cooked, meat only	145 gm	123
Shrimp	3 ounces, cooked	130
Heart, beef	3 ounces, cooked	230
Egg	1 yolk or 1 egg	250
Liver, beef, calf, hog, lamb	3 ounces, cooked	370
Kidney	3 ounces, cooked	680
Brains	3 ounces, raw	more than 1700

Source: U. S. Department of Agriculture

CAN YOU EAT TOO LITTLE FAT?

Perhaps it is possible to eat dangerously low amounts of fat if you're on a near-starvation diet, but the possibility is very remote for ordinary American eaters. Studies have shown that both adults and youngsters on a highly controlled synthetic diet of only 1 percent (in linoleic acid) showed no ill effects during a six-month to two-year trial. The fact is virtually no foods are totally absent of fat, so you are bound to get some fat if you eat at all. For example, blackberries have one fat gram per cup, as do dried beans. Nearly all fruits, vegetables, and grains have at least traces of fat, even lettuce. So it is impossible to eat a no-fat diet of ordinary foods and stay alive.

One question sometimes raised is: Will I get enough protein if I cut down on fatty foods? Protein deficiency has never been a problem in this country, except among the exceedingly undernourished. Most people get far more protein than they need, especially from high-fat animal products. But the notion you cannot eat a diet low in fat and consume enough protein, and other nutrients is a myth. Many low-fat dairy products, such as dry cottage cheese, yogurt, skim milk have high amounts of protein. Taking away their fat grams does not destroy their protein value. One cup of skim milk provides 20 percent of the adult recommended daily allowances for protein and has practically no fat. One cup of evaporated skim milk offers 40 percent of your daily protein requirement. One half cup of dry cottage cheese (with one gram of fat) provides 40 percent of your daily protein needs. Similarly, chicken and fish are high in protein and low in fat. Three ounces of crab meat has 35 percent of the daily protein needs and two grams of fat.*

Grains and vegetables contain small amounts of protein. The protein in these plant products is often termed "incomplete" because it lacks all the amino acids necessary to the body. However, as Frances Moore Lappe points out in her excellent book, *Diet for A Small Planet*, by combining certain foods, such as beans and rice, you can get a complete protein. She also notes that plant protein can be of quite high quality. She says when it comes to "net protein utilization" (the efficiency with which the body can use protein) rice and grains rank relatively high. For example, whole rice is on a par with meat in "net protein utilization." Experts generally say that if you're eating enough calories, you're probably getting enough protein.

What about other nutrients, such as Vitamin A, which is fat-soluble? It is true that the fat in milk and butter carries high amounts of vitamin A, and that skim milk

---

*For a more comprehensive overview of the nutrients in various foods, see *Brand Name Nutrition Counter* by Jean Carper, Bantam Books.

does not have significant amounts of vitamin A. However, that's not a problem if you eat a variety of other low-fat foods. One cup of carrots has two to three times the recommended daily allowance of vitamin A, as does one cup of pumpkin, spinach, or sweet potatoes. Grains do not ordinarily contain high levels of vitamin A, but most processed cereals on the market do because they are vitamin fortified. A serving of most cereals contains from 25 to 100 percent of the required vitamin A per day, as well as similar levels of several other nutrients.

Certainly a diet low in fat, like other type diets, could be dangerously deficient in nutrients if you do not eat a *variety* of foods. But, if you do that, you are *more* likely to get the necessary nutrients on a low-fat diet than on a high-fat one, according to Senator McGovern's nutrition committee. The reason, as Senator McGovern's committee concluded, is that fats are "relatively poor sources of micronutrients, particularly in view of the calories they induce." In other words, per calorie, fatty foods have fewer nutrients; that is, they have a lower nutrient density. When you're trying to keep your weight down, you especially need to maximize the nutrients per calorie. One way to do it is by eating low-fat foods.

According to McGovern's committee, when you eat a high-fat diet you often replace highly nutritious carbohydrates with less nutritious fatty calories. Thus, the committee said: "Increased consumption of fruit, vegetables and whole grains is important with respect to supplying adequate amounts of vitamins and minerals and micronutrients"—trace minerals, such as chromium and selenium which are vital to health.

One other pointer: It is better to eat *whole* grain breads and cereals and brown rice, simply because they provide more nutrients than highly processed white flour products and white rice. This is equally true whether you are on a low-fat or high-fat diet.

A diet low in fat can be a vegetarian diet, but it need not be. You can still eat meat, just less of it, and it should be lean, well-trimmed of fat. For example, heart and cancer specialist Dr. Wynder says he eats red meat only once a week. You can also eat chicken, turkey, and fish, all of which are low in fat, as long as they are not drenched in sauces or fried.

On the other hand, many people in the country are becoming vegetarians. The late anthropologist Margaret Mead predicted that within fifty years the country would be largely vegetarian. Such a diet by necessity is a low-fat one and can be perfectly healthful if you take precautions to make sure you get all the necessary protein, vitamins and minerals, notably B-12 and iron.

Though vitamin mineral pills are never a substitute for food, it may be necessary to supplement your diet with these nutrients. It is almost impossible, for example, for women of menstrual age, even on conventional high-fat diets, to get enough iron, and some nutritional experts now recommend extra iron for women as a matter of course.

ONE CAUTION: Do not cut down on fat by totally restricting yourself to only a few foods or one food, such as rice. This could be dangerous because it deprives your body of essential nutrients. If you have any doubts, consult your physician. This particularly applies to infants. Although babies, like others, do not need an excessively high-fat diet, consult your physician before putting an infant on a restrictive diet of any kind. Depriving children of vital nutrients at an early age could produce long-term damage. Also, being on a low-fat diet does not mean you can never eat high-fat foods. You can, as long as you balance them out with low-fat foods. Remember, it is not one or two fatty foods that matter; it is the *total* amount of fat in your diet that counts.

TIPS FOR LOW-FAT COOKING

- Sauté vegetables in water or a fat-free stock instead of fat.
- Use skim milk, buttermilk, low-fat yogurt, or uncreamed cottage cheese to make salad dressings instead of salad oil.

- Make white sauce with nonfat milk instead of whole milk or cream and omit the butter.
- Drain all excess oil from canned tuna fish and sardines before using.
- Trim meat of all visible fat before cooking.
- Remove skin from turkey and chicken before eating.
- If you make stock from fatty foods, chill it and skim the fat off when it is solid.
- Substitute skim milk for whole milk.

COUNTING FAT GRAMS TO LOSE WEIGHT

Counting fat grams is one of the easiest ways to take off pounds and probably the safest. For you are not depriving yourself of vital nutrients; fat is fairly low in nutrients. And because low-fat foods are often bulky, you don't suffer hunger pangs because they fill you up. The fact is that by cutting down on fat grams, you automatically cut back severely on calories. As noted previously, the calories in many fattening foods come from fat grams. Dr. George B. Vahouny, a biochemist at George Washington University, has suggested that counting fat grams may well become the accepted pattern for dieting in the near future.

If you're an average American now eating more than 40 percent of your calories in fat, and you cut back to 20 or 10 percent, you're bound to lose weight. Let's say you want to go on a 1500 calorie a day diet. You could eat 150 calories—or 10 percent of 1500—a day in fat, which would mean no more than 17 grams of fat per day. (9 calories per 1 fat gram). Experience in Great Britain has shown that restricting yourself to even 250 calories per day from fat (or about 28 grams of fat) will cause considerable weight loss in most people. The glory of such a diet is that once you restrict the amount of fat you eat, you can eat almost as much of everything else as you can physically consume—and still lose weight. A couple of exceptions: alcohol and sugar, which are high in calories.

Remember complex carbohydrates (typically called starchy foods) are good for you. And these are usually what you'll be eating more of when you cut down on fats. Further, a relatively low-fat diet, unlike many other diets, is one that you can follow with great safety and in good health for the rest of your life.

Abbreviations

diam	diameter
fl	fluid
in	inch
lb	pound
med	medium
oz	ounce
pkg	package
swt	sweetened
tbsp	tablespoon
tsp	teaspoon
unswt	unsweetened
w	with
wo	without

Appetizers

Frozen	FAT GRAMS	PERCENT OF CALORIES FROM FAT
Cheese straws: 1 piece / **Durkee**	2	60–70
Frankfurter: 1 piece / **Durkee** Franks-n-Blankets	4	80–90
Puff pastry: 1 piece		
Beef puffs / **Durkee**	5	80–90
Cheese puffs / **Durkee**	6	80–90
Chicken puffs / **Durkee**	5	80–90
Chicken liver puffs / **Durkee**	5	80–90
Shrimp puffs / **Durkee**	4	70–80

Baby Food

A note: Cereals, fruits and vegetables (unless they have butter, sauces or meat added) are universally low in fat. However, you will note that the fat content varies ever so slightly among some similar products, depending on the baby food company. The small differences occur generally because of the method of analysis or the way the figures are reported. For example, one company may round off .5 grams of fat to 1 gram and .4 to zero. Such small differences are insignificant when choosing a product.

BAKED GOODS

	FAT GRAMS	PERCENT OF CALORIES FROM FAT
Biscuits, teething: 1 piece / Gerber	.5	0–10
Cookies, animal shaped:		
1 cookie / Gerber	1	20–30
Cookies, arrowroot: 1 cookie / Gerber	1	20–30
Pretzels: 1 pretzel / Gerber	0	0–10
Toast, zwieback: 1 piece / Gerber	1	20–30

STRAINED BABY FOODS

Cereal: 1 jar

High protein w applesauce and bananas / Gerber	1	0–10
Mixed w apples and bananas / Heinz	0	0–10

3

	FAT GRAMS	PERCENT OF CALORIES FROM FAT
Mixed w applesauce and bananas / **Gerber**	1	0–10
Mixed w fruit / **Beech-Nut**	0	0–10
Oatmeal w apples and bananas / **Heinz**	1	0–10
Oatmeal w applesauce and bananas / **Gerber**	1	0–10
Oatmeal w fruit / **Beech-Nut**	0	0–10
Rice w apples and bananas / **Heinz**	0	0–10
Rice w applesauce and bananas / **Gerber**	0	0–10

Cereal, dry: ½ oz

Barley / **Gerber**	1	10–20
Barley / **Heinz**	0	0–10
High protein / **Gerber**	1	10–20
High protein / **Heinz**	0	0–10
High protein w apple and orange / **Gerber**	1	10–20
Mixed / **Gerber**	1	10–20
Mixed / **Heinz**	0	0–10
Mixed w banana / **Gerber**	1	10–20
Oatmeal / **Gerber**	1	10–20
Oatmeal / **Heinz**	1	0–10
Oatmeal w banana / **Gerber**	1	10–20
Rice / **Gerber**	1	10–20
Rice / **Heinz**	0	0–10
Rice w banana / **Gerber**	1	10–20

Formula, meat base: 2 tbsp / Gerber

Infant Formula	2	40–50

Fruits and Desserts: 1 jar

Apple betty / **Beech-Nut**	0	0–10
Apple blueberry / **Gerber**	1	0–10

	FAT GRAMS	PERCENT OF CALORIES FROM FAT
Apple raspberry / Gerber	1	0–10
Apples and apricots / Beech-Nut	0	0–10
Apples and cranberries w tapioca / Heinz	0	0–10
Apples and pears / Heinz	0	0–10
Applesauce / Beech-Nut	0	0–10
Applesauce / Gerber	1	0–10
Applesauce / Heinz	0	0–10
Applesauce and apricots / Gerber	0	0–10
Applesauce and apricots / Heinz	0	0–10
Applesauce and cherries / Beech-Nut	0	0–10
Applesauce w pineapple / Gerber	1	1–10
Applesauce and raspberries / Beech-Nut	0	0–10
Apricots w tapioca / Beech-Nut	0	0–10
Apricots w tapioca / Gerber	1	0–10
Apricots w tapioca / Heinz	0	0–10
Bananas and pineapple / Beech-Nut	0	0–10
Bananas w pineapple and tapioca / Gerber	1	0–10
Bananas and pineapple w tapioca / Heinz	0	0–10
Bananas w tapioca / Beech-Nut	0	0–10
Bananas w tapioca / Gerber	1	0–10
Bananas w tapioca / Heinz	0	0–10
Cottage cheese w pineapple / Gerber	1	0–10
Dutch apple dessert / Gerber	1	0–10
Dutch apple dessert / Heinz	1	0–10
Fruit dessert / Gerber	1	0–10
Fruit dessert / Heinz	0	0–10
Fruit dessert w tapioca / Beech-Nut	0	0–10
Hawaiian delight / Gerber	1	0–10

	FAT GRAMS	PERCENT OF CALORIES FROM FAT
Orange-pineapple dessert / **Beech-Nut**	0	0–10
Peach cobbler / **Gerber**	0	0–10
Peach cobbler / **Heinz**	0	0–10
Peach melba / **Beech-Nut**	0	0–10
Peaches / **Beech-Nut**	0	0–10
Peaches / **Gerber**	0	0–10
Peaches / **Heinz**	0	0–10
Pears / **Beech-Nut**	0	0–10
Pears / **Gerber**	1	0–10
Pears / **Heinz**	0	0–10
Pears and pineapple / **Beech-Nut**	0	0–10
Pears and pineapple / **Gerber**	0	0–10
Pears and pineapple / **Heinz**	0	0–10
Pineapple dessert / **Beech-Nut**	0	0–10
Plums w tapioca / **Beech-Nut**	0	0–10
Plums w tapioca / **Gerber**	1	0–10
Plums w tapioca / **Heinz**	0	0–10
Prunes w tapioca / **Beech-Nut**	0	0–10
Prunes w tapioca / **Gerber**	1	0–10
Prunes w tapioca / **Heinz**	0	0–10
Pudding		
Banana / **Heinz**	2	10–20
Cherry vanilla / **Gerber**	1	0–10
Custard / **Heinz**	4	30–40
Custard, apple / **Beech-Nut**	1.5	20–30
Custard, chocolate / **Gerber**	2	10–15
Custard, vanilla / **Gerber**	3	20–30
Orange / **Gerber**	1	0–10
Orange / **Heinz**	0	0–10
Tutti-frutti / **Heinz**	0	0–10
Yogurt, mixed fruit / **Beech-Nut**	0	0–10
Yogurt, peach-apple / **Beech-Nut**	0	0–10
Yogurt, pineapple / **Beech-Nut**	0	0–10

	FAT GRAMS	PERCENT OF CALORIES FROM FAT
Juices: 1 can		
Apple / **Beech-Nut**	0	0–10
Apple / **Gerber**	0	0–10
Apple / **Heinz**	0	0–10
Apple-cherry / **Beech-Nut**	0	0–10
Apple-cherry / **Gerber**	1	0–10
Apple-grape / **Beech-Nut**	0	0–10
Apple-grape / **Gerber**	0	0–10
Apple-grape / **Heinz**	0	0–10
Apple-peach / **Gerber**	0	0–10
Apple-pineapple / **Heinz**	0	0–10
Apple-plum / **Gerber**	0	0–10
Apple-prune / **Heinz**	0	0–10
Apricot / **Heinz**	0	0–10
Cherry / **Heinz**	0	0–10
Mixed fruit / **Beech-Nut**	0	0–10
Mixed fruit / **Gerber**	1	0–10
Orange / **Beech-Nut**	0	0–10
Orange / **Gerber**	1	0–10
Orange / **Heinz**	0	0–10
Orange-apple / **Beech-Nut**	0	0–10
Orange-apple / **Gerber**	1	0–10
Orange-apple-banana / **Gerber**	1	0–10
Orange-apple-banana drink / **Heinz**	0	0–10
Orange-apricot / **Gerber**	0	0–10
Orange-banana / **Beech-Nut**	0	0–10
Orange-pineapple / **Beech-Nut**	0	0–10
Orange-pineapple / **Gerber**	0	0–10
Orange-pineapple drink / **Heinz**	0	0–10
Prune-orange / **Beech-Nut**	0	0–10
Prune-orange / **Gerber**	0	0–10
Main Dishes: 1 jar		
Beef / **Beech-Nut**	7.3	50–60
Beef / **Beech-Nut** High Meat Dinner	7.7	50–60

	FAT GRAMS	PERCENT OF CALORIES FROM FAT
Beef / **Gerber**	5	40–50
Beef w beef hearts / **Gerber**	4	30–40
Beef and noodles / **Beech-Nut**	2.4	30–40
Beef and noodles w vegetables / **Gerber**	3	30–40
Beef w vegetables / **Gerber** High Meat Dinner	5	40–50
Cereal and egg yolks / **Gerber**	2	20–30
Cereal, egg yolks and bacon / **Beech-Nut**	6.7	50–60
Cereal and Eggs / **Heinz**	1	10–20
Chicken / **Beech-Nut**	5.8	40–50
Chicken / **Beech-Nut** High Meat Dinner	3.1	30–40
Chicken / **Gerber**	8	50–60
Chicken noodle / **Beech-Nut**	.6	0–10
Chicken and noodles / **Gerber**	2	20–30
Chicken w vegetables / **Beech-Nut**	.6	0–10
Chicken w vegetables / **Gerber** High Meat Dinner	5	40–50
Cottage cheese w bananas / **Heinz**	0	0–10
Cottage cheese w pineapple / **Gerber** High Meat Dinners	1	0–10
Cottage cheese w pineapple juice / **Beech-Nut**	.9	0–10
Egg yolks / **Gerber**	16	80–90
Egg yolks / **Heinz**	15	80–90
Grits w egg yolks / **Gerber**	3	30–40
Ham / **Beech-Nut**	7	50–60
Ham / **Beech-Nut** High Meat Dinner	8.6	50–60
Ham / **Gerber**	6	40–50
Ham w vegetables / **Gerber** High Meat Dinner	4	30–40
Lamb / **Beech-Nut**	7.4	50–60
Lamb / **Gerber**	4	30–40

	FAT GRAMS	PERCENT OF CALORIES FROM FAT
Liver, beef / **Gerber**	3	30–40
Macaroni and cheese / **Gerber**	3	30–40
Macaroni, tomato sauce, beef and bacon / **Beech-Nut**	2.4	10–20
Macaroni w tomatoes and beef / **Gerber**	1	10–20
Pork / **Gerber**	7	50–60
Soup, chicken, cream of / **Gerber**	3	30–40
Turkey / **Beech-Nut**	6.4	50–60
Turkey / **Beech-Nut** High Meat Dinner	6.1	50–60
Turkey / **Gerber**	8	50–60
Turkey and rice / **Beech-Nut**	1	10–20
Turkey and rice w vegetables / **Gerber**	3	30–40
Turkey w vegetables / **Gerber** High Meat Dinner	6	40–50
Veal / **Beech-Nut**	6.6	50–60
Veal / **Beech-Nut** High Meat Dinner	3.2	30–40
Veal / **Gerber**	4	40–50
Veal w vegetables / **Gerber** High Meat dinner	3	30–40
Vegetables and bacon / **Beech-Nut**	3.6	40–50
Vegetables and bacon / **Gerber**	5	40–50
Vegetables and beef / **Beech-Nut**	2.4	20–30
Vegetables and beef / **Gerber**	3	30–40
Vegetables and chicken / **Gerber**	2	30–40
Vegetables and ham / **Beech-Nut**	1.3	10–20
Vegetables and ham / **Gerber**	2	20–30
Vegetables and lamb / **Beech-Nut**	2.4	30–40
Vegetables and lamb / **Gerber**	3	30–40
Vegetables and liver / **Beech-Nut**	.4	0–10
Vegetables and liver / **Gerber**	1	10–20
Vegetables and turkey / **Gerber**	2	30–40

	FAT GRAMS	PERCENT OF CALORIES FROM FAT
Vegetables: 1 jar		
Beans, green / **Beech-Nut**	0	0–10
Beans, green / **Gerber**	0	0–10
Beans, green / **Heinz**	0	0–10
Beets / **Gerber**	0	0–10
Beets / **Heinz**	0	0–10
Carrots / **Beech-Nut**	0	0–10
Carrots / **Gerber**	0	0–10
Carrots / **Heinz**	0	0–10
Corn, creamed / **Beech-Nut**	.4	0–10
Corn, creamed / **Gerber**	1	0–10
Corn, creamed / **Heinz**	0	0–10
Garden vegetables / **Beech-Nut**	0	0–10
Garden vegetables / **Gerber**	1	10–20
Mixed / **Gerber**	1	10–20
Mixed / **Heinz**	1	10–20
Peas / **Beech-Nut**	.4	0–10
Peas / **Gerber**	1	0–10
Peas, creamed / **Heinz**	2.3	20–30
Spinach, creamed / **Gerber**	2	30–40
Squash / **Beech-Nut**	0	0–10
Squash / **Gerber**	0	0–10
Squash / **Heinz**	0	0–10
Sweet potatoes / **Beech-Nut**	0	0–10
Sweet potatoes / **Gerber**	0	0–10
Sweet potatoes / **Heinz**	0	0–10

JUNIOR BABY FOODS

Cereal: 1 jar		
Mixed w applesauce and bananas / **Gerber**	1	0–10
Oatmeal w applesauce and bananas / **Gerber**	2	0–10
Rice cereal w mixed fruit / **Gerber**	1	0–10

	FAT GRAMS	PERCENT OF CALORIES FROM FAT
Fruits and Desserts: 1 jar		
Apple betty / **Beech-Nut**	0	0–10
Apple-blueberry / **Gerber**	1	0–10
Apple-raspberry / **Gerber**	1	0–10
Apples and apricots / **Beech-Nut**	0	0–10
Apples and cranberries / **Heinz**	0	0–10
Apples and pears / **Heinz**	0	0–10
Applesauce / **Beech-Nut**	0	0–10
Applesauce / **Gerber**	0	0–10
Applesauce / **Heinz**	0	0–10
Applesauce and apricots / **Gerber**	1	0–10
Applesauce and apricots / **Heinz**	0	0–10
Applesauce and cherries / **Beech-Nut**	0	0–10
Applesauce w pineapple / **Gerber**	1	0–10
Applesauce and raspberries / **Beech-Nut**	0	0–10
Apricots w tapioca / **Beech-Nut**	0	0–10
Apricots w tapioca / **Gerber**	1	0–10
Apricots w tapioca / **Heinz**	1	0–10
Banana dessert / **Beech-Nut**	0	0–10
Bananas w pineapple and tapioca / **Beech-Nut**	0	0–10
Bananas w pineapple and tapioca / **Gerber**	1	0–10
Bananas w tapioca / **Gerber**	1	0–10
Cottage cheese w pineapple / **Beech-Nut**	1.5	0–10
Cottage cheese w pineapple / **Gerber**	2	0–10
Dutch apple dessert / **Gerber**	2	0–10
Fruit dessert / **Gerber**	1	0–10
Fruit dessert / **Heinz**	0	0–10
Fruit dessert w tapioca / **Beech-Nut**	0	0–10
Hawaiian delight / **Gerber**	1	0–10

	FAT GRAMS	PERCENT OF CALORIES FROM FAT
Peach cobbler / Gerber	1	0–10
Peach cobbler / Heinz	0	0–10
Peach melba / Beech-Nut	0	0–10
Peaches / Beech-Nut	0	0–10
Peaches / Gerber	1	0–10
Peaches / Heinz	1	0–10
Pears / Beech-Nut	0	0–10
Pears / Gerber	1	0–10
Pears / Heinz	0	0–10
Pears and pineapple / Beech-Nut	0	0–10
Pears and pineapple / Gerber	1	0–10
Pears and pineapple / Heinz	0	0–10
Pineapple-orange dessert / Heinz	0	0–10
Plums w tapioca / Beech-Nut	0	0–10
Plums w tapioca / Gerber	1	0–10
Plums w tapioca / Heinz	0	0–10
Prunes w tapioca / Beech-Nut	0	0–10
Prunes w tapioca / Gerber	1	0–10
Prunes w tapioca / Heinz	0	0–10
Pudding		
Cherry vanilla / Gerber	1	0–10
Custard / Heinz	6	20–30
Custard, apple / Beech-Nut	2.6	10–20
Custard, cholocate / Gerber	4	10–20
Custard, vanilla / Gerber	1	0–10
Tropical fruit dessert / Beech-Nut	0	0–10
Tutti-frutti / Heinz	1	0–10
Yogurt, mixed fruit / Beech-Nut	0	0–10
Yogurt, peach-apple / Beech-Nut	0	0–10
Yogurt, pineapple / Beech-Nut	0	0–10

Main Dishes: 1 jar

Beef / Beech-Nut	7.3	50–60
Beef / Beech-Nut High Meat Dinner	7.7	50–60
Beef / Gerber	4	30–40

	FAT GRAMS	PERCENT OF CALORIES FROM FAT
Beef and noodles / **Beech-Nut**	4.1	30–40
Beef and egg noodles w vegetables / **Gerber**	4	30–40
Beef and rice w tomato sauce / **Gerber** Toddler Meals	5	30–40
Beef stew / **Gerber** Toddler Meals	2	10–20
Beef w vegetables / **Gerber** High Meat Dinner	5	40–50
Cereal and egg yolk / **Gerber**	4	30–40
Cereal, egg yolks and bacon / **Beech-Nut**	11.5	50–60
Cereal and eggs / **Heinz**	2	10–20
Chicken / **Beech-Nut**	5.8	40–50
Chicken / **Beech-Nut** High Meat Dinner	3.1	30–40
Chicken / **Gerber**	10	60–70
Chicken noodle / **Beech-Nut**	1.1	10–20
Chicken and noodles / **Gerber**	3	20–30
Chicken stew / **Gerber** Toddler Meals	7	40–50
Chicken sticks / **Gerber**	10	60–70
Chicken w vegetables / **Beech-Nut**	.6	0–10
Chicken w vegetables / **Gerber**	8	50–60
Cottage cheese w bananas / **Heinz**	0	0–10
Ham / **Beech-Nut** High Meat Dinner	8.6	60–70
Ham / **Gerber**	7	50–60
Ham casserole w green beans and potatoes / **Gerber** Toddler Meals	6	30–40
Ham w vegetables / **Gerber** High Meat Dinner	4	30–40
Lamb / **Beech-Nut**	7.4	50–60
Lamb / **Gerber**	4	30–40
Lasagna, beef / **Gerber** Toddler Meals	4	20–30

	FAT GRAMS	PERCENT OF CALORIES FROM FAT
Macaroni and beef / **Beech-Nut**	3.8	20–30
Macaroni and cheese / **Gerber**	4	20–30
Macaroni, tomato and beef / **Gerber**	2	10–20
Meat sticks / **Gerber**	10	60–70
Peas, split w ham / **Gerber**	3	10–20
Peas, split w vegetables and ham / **Beech-Nut**	2.3	10–20
Spaghetti, tomato sauce and beef / **Beech-Nut**	3.6	20–30
Spaghetti w tomato sauce and beef / **Gerber**	3	10–20
Spaghetti and meat balls / **Gerber** Toddler Meals	2	10–20
Turkey / **Beech-Nut**	6.4	50–60
Turkey / **Beech-Nut** High Meat Dinner	6.1	40–50
Turkey / **Gerber**	7	50–60
Turkey and rice / **Beech-Nut**	1.1	10–20
Turkey and rice w vegetables / **Gerber**	4	30–40
Turkey sticks / **Gerber**	10	70–80
Turkey w vegetables / **Gerber**	7	50–60
Veal / **Beech-Nut**	6.6	50–60
Veal / **Beech-Nut** High Meat Dinner	3.2	30–40
Veal / **Gerber**	4	30–40
Veal w vegetables / **Gerber**	4	30–40
Vegetables and bacon / **Beech-Nut**	5.8	30–40
Vegetables and bacon / **Gerber**	10	50–60
Vegetables and beef / **Beech-Nut**	3.6	20–30
Vegetables and beef / **Gerber**	4	30–40
Vegetables and chicken / **Gerber**	3	20–30
Vegetables and ham / **Gerber**	4	30–40
Vegetables and lamb / **Beech-Nut**	3.8	30–40
Vegetables and lamb / **Gerber**	4	30–40
Vegetables and liver / **Beech-Nut**	.4	0–10

	FAT GRAMS	PERCENT OF CALORIES FROM FAT
Vegetables and liver / **Gerber**	1	10–20
Vegetables and turkey / **Gerber**	3	20–30
Vegetables and turkey casserole / **Gerber** Toddler Meals	6	30–40

Vegetables: 1 jar

Beans, green / **Beech-Nut**	0	0–10
Beans, green, creamed / **Gerber**	1	0–10
Carrots / **Beech-Nut**	0	0–10
Carrots / **Gerber**	1	0–10
Carrots / **Heinz**	0	0–10
Corn, creamed / **Beech-Nut**	.6	0–10
Corn, creamed / **Gerber**	1	0–10
Corn, creamed / **Heinz**	1	0–10
Mixed / **Gerber**	1	0–10
Mixed / **Heinz**	0	0–10
Peas / **Beech-Nut**	.6	0–10
Peas, creamed / **Heinz**	4	20–30
Spinach, creamed / **Gerber**	3	20–30
Squash / **Beech-Nut**	0	0–10
Squash / **Gerber**	1	0–10
Sweet potatoes / **Beech-Nut**	0	0–10
Sweet potatoes / **Gerber**	0	0–10
Sweet potatoes / **Heinz**	0	0–10

Baking Powder

No fat

Beer, Ale, Malt Liquor

No fat

Biscuits

	FAT GRAMS	PERCENT OF CALORIES FROM FAT
Refrigerator: 1 biscuit		
Ballard Oven Ready	.5	0–10
1869 Brand	5	40–50
Hungry Jack Butter Tastin	4.5	40–50
Hungry Jack Flaky	4.5	40–50
Pillsbury Country Style	.5	0–10
Pillsbury Prize	2.5	30–40
Baking powder / **1869 Brand**	5	40–50
Baking powder, prebaked /		
1869 Brand	5	40–50
Baking powder / **Tenderflake** Dinner	2.5	30–40
Buttermilk		
1869 Brand	5	40–50
1869 Brand, prebaked	5.5	40–50
Hungry Jack Extra Rich	3	40–50
Hungry Jack Flaky	2	20–30
Hungry Jack Fluffy	5	40–50
Pillsbury	.5	0–10
Pillsbury Big Country	2.5	20–30
Pillsbury Extra Lights	1	10–20
Tenderflake Dinner	2	30–40
Corn bread / **Pillsbury**	4.5	40–50

Bread

	FAT GRAMS	PERCENT OF CALORIES FROM FAT
1 slice unless noted		
Brown, plain, canned: ½-in slice / **B & M**	trace	0–10
Brown, raisin, canned: ½-in slice / **B & M**	.3	0–10
Cinnamon raisin / **Thomas'**	1	10–20
Corn and molasses / **Pepperidge Farm**	.5	0–10
French: 1 oz / **Pepperidge Farm**	1	10–20
French: 1 oz / **Wonder**	1	10–20
Garlic, frozen / **Stouffer's**	4	40–50
Gluten / **Thomas'** Glutogen	.5	10–20
Hollywood Light	1	10–20
Hollywood Dark	1	10–20
Honey bran / **Pepperidge Farm**	1	10–20
Honey Wheatberry / **Arnold**	1	10–20
Honey Wheatberry / **Pepperidge Farm**	1	10–20
Italian: 1 oz / **Pepperidge Farm**	1.5	10–20
Meal / **Roman** Meal	1	10–20
Naturél / **Arnold**	1	10–20
Oatmeal / **Pepperidge Farm**	1	10–20
Profile Dark	1.5	10–20
Profile Light	1	10–20
Protein / **Thomas'** Protogen	.5	10–20
Pumpernickel / **Arnold**	.5	0–10
Pumpernickel / **Pepperidge Farm** Family	1	10–20
Pumpernickel / **Pepperidge Farm** Party	.5	10–20
Raisin / **Arnold** Tea	1	10–20
Raisin / **Pepperidge Farm**	1.5	10–20

	FAT GRAMS	PERCENT OF CALORIES FROM FAT
Rye		
Arnold Melba Thin	.5	0–10
Arnold Soft	.5	10–20
Pepperidge Farm Family	1	10–20
Pepperidge Farm Party	.2	10–20
Wonder	1	10–20
Jewish, seeded / **Arnold**	1	10–20
Jewish / **Pepperidge Farm**	1	10–20
Seedless / **Pepperidge Farm**	1	10–20
Sourdough / **DiCarlo**	.5	0–10
Wheat		
Arnold American Granary	1	10–20
Arnold Bran'nola	1.5	10–20
Arnold Brick Oven Whole Wheat (small family)	1.5	10–20
Arnold Brick OvenWhole Wheat 16 oz	1.5	20–30
Arnold Whole Wheat 32 oz	2	20–30
Arnold Melba Thin Whole Wheat	1	20–30
Fresh Horizons	.5	0–10
Home Pride Butter Top Wheat	1.5	10–20
Home Pride Wheatberry	1	10–20
Light Wheat Fiber	.5	0–10
Pepperidge Farm 1½ lb	1.5	10–20
Pepperidge Farm Whole Wheat 1 lb	1.5	10–20
Pepperidge Farm Very Thin Whole Wheat	1	20–30
Pritikin 100% Whole Wheat	.5	0–10
Thomas' Whole Wheat	1	10–20
Wonder	1	10–20
Wonder Whole Wheat	1	10–20
Cracked wheat / **Pepperidge Farm**	1	10–20
Cracked wheat / **Wonder**	1	10–20
Wheat germ / **Pepperidge Farm**	.5	0–10
Sprouted wheat / **Pepperidge Farm**	1	10–20

	FAT GRAMS	PERCENT OF CALORIES FROM FAT
White		
Arnold Brick Oven 32 oz	1.5	10–20
Arnold Brick Oven 16 oz	1	10–20
Arnold Brick Oven (small family)	1	10–20
Arnold Country	1.5	10–20
Arnold Hearthstone Country	1.5	10–20
Arnold Melba Thin	1	20–30
Fresh Horizons	.5	0–10
Hearthstone	1.5	10–20
Hillbilly	1	10–20
Home Pride Butter Top White	1.5	10–20
Light White Fiber	.5	0–10
Mrs. Karl's	1	10–20
Pepperidge Farm Family	1.5	10–20
Pepperidge Farm Sandwich	1	10–20
Pepperidge Farm Thin Sliced	1.5	10–20
Pepperidge Farm Toasting	1	10–20
Pepperidge Farm Unsliced: 1 oz	2	20–30
Pepperidge Farm Very Thin	.5	10–20
Weight Watchers	.5	10–20
Wonder	1	10–20
Refrigerator, to bake / **Pillsbury** Hotloaf	2	10–20

BREAD CRUMBS

Bread crumbs: 1 cup / Contadina	3	0–10

BREAD MIXES

Prepared: 1 loaf unless noted

Applesauce spice / **Pillsbury**	48	20–30
Apricot nut / **Pillsbury**	32	10–20
Banana / **Pillsbury**	48	20–30
Blueberry nut / **Pillsbury**	32	10–20
Cherry nut / **Pillsbury**	48	20–30

	FAT GRAMS	PERCENT OF CALORIES FROM FAT
Corn: 1 pkg / **Aunt Jemima** Easy Mix	42	20–30
Corn: 1 pkg / **Pillsbury**	32	20–30
Cranberry / **Pillsbury**	48	20–30
Date / **Pillsbury**	32	10–20
Nut / **Pillsbury**	64	30–40
Oatmeal raisin / **Pillsbury**	48	20–30

BREADSTICKS

1 stick

Onion / **Stella D'Oro**	1.1	20–30
Plain / **Stella D'Oro**	1.2	20–30
Plain / **Stella D'Oro Dietetic**	1.2	20–30
Sesame / **Stella D'Oro**	2.2	30–40
Sesame / **Stella D'Oro Dietetic**	2.5	30–40

CROUTONS

Artificial bacon: ¼ cup / **Bel Air**	1	20–30
Cheddar cheese: 1 oz / **Pepperidge Farm**	5	30–40
Cheese and garlic: ¼ cup / **Bel Air**	2	30–40
Cheese-garlic: 1 oz / **Pepperidge Farm**	7	40–50
Garlic: ¼ cup / **Bel Air**	1	20–30
Italian cheese: ¼ cup / **Bel Air**	2	30–40
Onion-garlic: 1 oz / **Pepperidge Farm**	6	30–40
Plain: ¼ cup / **Bel Air**	0	0–10
Plain: 1 oz / **Pepperidge Farm**	5	30–40
Seasoned: ¼ cup / **Bel Air**	1	20–30
Seasoned: 1 oz / **Pepperidge Farm**	5	30–40

Butter and Margarine

	FAT GRAMS	PERCENT OF CALORIES FROM FAT
Butter		
Regular: ½ cup (¼ lb stick)	91.9	100
1 tbsp	11.5	100
Whipped: ½ cup	61.2	100
1 tbsp	7.6	100
Margarine		
Regular and Soft: 1 tbsp		
Blue Bonnet	11	100
Blue Bonnet Diet	6	100
Blue Bonnet Soft	11	100
Chiffon Soft	11	100
Chiffon Stick	11	100
Coldbrook	11	100
Coldbrook Soft	11	100
Dalewood	11	100
Empress	11	100
Empress Soft	11	100
Fleischmann's	11	100
Fleischmann's Diet	6	100
Fleischmann's Parve	11	100
Fleischmann's Soft	11	100
Holiday	11	100
Mazola	11	100
Meadowlake	11	100
Mrs. Filbert's	11	100
Mrs. Filbert's Soft	11	100
Nucoa	11	100
Nucoa Soft	10	100

	FAT GRAMS	PERCENT OF CALORIES FROM FAT
Parkay	11	100
Swift Allsweet	11	100
Whipped: 1 tbsp		
Blue Bonnet		
Whipped stick and soft	7	100
Chiffon Soft	7	100
Fleischmann's Soft	7	100
Mrs. Filbert's Soft	8	100
Spread: 1 tbsp		
Blue Bonnet	8	100
Coldbrook	8	100
Fleischmann's	8	100
Imitation: 1 tbsp		
Mazola diet	5.6	100
Mrs. Filbert's diet soft	6	100
Parkay diet	6	100
Weight Watchers	6	100

STUFFING MIXES

	FAT GRAMS	PERCENT OF CALORIES FROM FAT
Chicken & Herb: 1 oz / **Pepperidge Farm** Pan Style	1	0–10
Chicken-flavored, prepared w butter: ½ cup / **Stove Top**	9	40–50
Chicken-flavored, prepared: ½ cup cooked w butter / **Uncle Ben's** Stuff'n Such	9.6	40–50
½ cup cooked wo butter / **Uncle Ben's** Stuff'n Such	1.1	0–10
Corn bread: 1 oz / **Pepperidge Farm**	1	0–10
Cornbread, prepared w butter: ½ cup / **Stove Top**	8	40–50
Corn bread, prepared: ½ cup cooked w butter / **Uncle Ben's** Stuff'n Such	9.5	40–50
½ cup cooked wo butter / **Uncle Ben's** Stuff'n Such	.9	0–10

	FAT GRAMS	PERCENT OF CALORIES FROM FAT
Cube: 1 oz / **Pepperidge Farm**	1	10–20
Sage: ½ cup cooked w butter /		
Uncle Ben's Stuff'n Such	9.5	40–50
½ cup cooked wo butter /		
Uncle Ben's Stuff'n Such	1	0–10
Seasoned: 1 oz / **Pepperidge Farm**	1	0–10
Pork-flavored, mix, prepared w		
butter: ½ cup / **Stove Top**	9	40–50
w rice, prepared w butter:		
½ cup / **Stove Top**	9	40–50

---

*Pepperidge Farm figures are for dry mix as packaged. Adding fat, such as butter, will increase the fat content.

Cakes

FROZEN DESSERT CAKES

	FAT GRAMS	PERCENT OF CALORIES FROM FAT
1 whole cake unless noted		
Banana / **Pepperidge Farm**	48	30–40
Banana / **Sara Lee**	55.2	30–40
Banana nut layer / **Sara Lee**	104	50–60
Black Forest / **Sara Lee**	74.4	40–50
Boston creme / **Pepperidge Farm**	40	30–40
Cheesecake		
Large / **Sara Lee**	79.8	50–60
Small / **Sara Lee**	48	50–60
Mrs. Smith's	54	40–50
Cherry cream / **Sara Lee**	57.6	40–50
French cream / **Sara Lee**	141.6	50–60
Strawberry cream / **Sara Lee**	58.2	40–50
Strawberry French cream / **Sara Lee**	117.6	50–60
Chocolate		
Pepperidge Farm	52	30–40
Sara Lee	71.2	40–50
Double layer / **Sara Lee**	99.2	50–60
'n cream layer / **Sara Lee**	99.2	50–60
Bavarian / **Sara Lee**	161.6	60–70
Fudge / **Pepperidge Farm**	90	40–50

25

	FAT GRAMS	PERCENT OF CALORIES FROM FAT
Fudge / **Pepperidge Farm**		
Half Cakes	45	40–50
German / **Pepperidge Farm**	60	30–40
German / **Sara Lee**	90.4	60–70
Coconut / **Pepperidge Farm**	90	40–50
Coconut / **Pepperidge Farm**		
Half Cakes	45	40–50
Coffee cake		
Almond / **Sara Lee**	71.2	40–50
Pecan, large / **Sara Lee**	73.6	40–50
Pecan, small / **Sara Lee**	42.4	40–50
Streusel, cinnamon / **Sara Lee**	68.8	50–60
Streusel, large, butter / **Sara Lee**	85.6	50–60
Coffee ring, almond / **Sara Lee**	67.2	50–60
Coffee ring, blueberry / **Sara Lee**	49.6	40–50
Coffee ring, maple crunch /		
Sara Lee	76	50–60
Coffee ring, raspberry / **Sara Lee**	56	40–50
Crumbcake		
Blueberry / **Sara Lee**	6.3	30–40
Blueberry / **Stouffer's**	8	30–40
Chocolate chip / **Stouffer's**	12	40–50
French / **Sara Lee**	6.8	30–40
French / **Stouffer's**	8	30–40
Cupcake		
Chocolate / **Sara Lee**	8.7	30–40
Chocolate, double / **Sara Lee**	9.1	40–50
Cream-filled / **Stouffer's**	11	40–50
Yellow / **Sara Lee**	6.8	30–40
Yellow / **Stouffer's**	8	30–40
Devil's food / **Pepperidge Farm**	80	40–50
Devil's food / **Sara Lee**	79.2	40–50
Golden / **Pepperidge Farm**		
Half Cakes	45	40–50
Golden / **Sara Lee**	62.4	30–40
Golden layer / **Pepperidge Farm**	90	40–50

	FAT GRAMS	PERCENT OF CALORIES FROM FAT
Lemon Bavarian / **Sara Lee**	154.4	60–70
Lemon coconut / **Pepperidge Farm**	44	30–40
Mandarin orange layer / **Sara Lee**	84	40–50
Pound Cake		
Sara Lee	66	40–50
Stouffer's / 1 oz	8	50–60
Apple nut / **Pepperidge Farm**		
Old Fashioned	50	30–40
Banana nut / **Sara Lee**	56	40–50
Butter / **Pepperidge Farm**		
Old Fashioned	70	40–50
Carrot / **Pepperidge Farm**		
Old Fashioned	90	50–60
Chocolate / **Pepperidge Farm**		
Old Fashioned	70	40–50
Chocolate / **Sara Lee**	80	50–60
Chocolate swirl / **Sara Lee**	57	30–40
Family size / **Sara Lee**	102	40–50
Home style / **Sara Lee**	59	40–50
Raisin / **Sara Lee**	58	40–50
Orange cake / **Sara Lee**	63.2	40–50
Cherry shortcake / **Mrs. Smith's**	108	40–50
Strawberry shortcake / **Sara Lee**	72.8	40–50
Strawberry shortcake / **Mrs. Smith's**	108	50–60
Strawberry 'n cream layer / **Sara Lee**	88.8	40–50
Vanilla / **Pepperidge Farm**	80	30–40
Walnut layer / **Sara Lee**	104	50–60

MIXES

**Prepared according to pkg directions:
1 whole cake**

Angel food / **Betty Crocker**	0	0
Angel food / **Betty Crocker** One-Step	0	0
Angel food / **Duncan Hines**	0	0
Angel food / **Pillsbury**	0	0

	FAT GRAMS	PERCENT OF CALORIES FROM FAT
Angel food, chocolate / **Betty Crocker**	0	0
Angel food, confetti / **Betty Crocker**	0	0
Angel food, lemon custard / **Betty Crocker**	0	0
Angel food, raspberry / **Pillsbury**	0	0
Angel food, strawberry / **Betty Crocker**	0	0
Apple raisin / **Duncan Hines**	60	20–30
Apple raisin, spicy / **Duncan Hines** Moist and Easy	36	20–30
Applesauce raisin / **Betty Crocker** Snackin' Cake	54	20–30
Banana / **Betty Crocker**	156	40–50
Banana / **Duncan Hines** Supreme	60	20–30
Banana / **Pillsbury Plus**	144	40–50
Banana Nut / **Duncan Hines** Moist and Easy	63	30–40
Banana walnut / **Betty Crocker** Snackin' Cake	63	30–40
Bundt cake		
Chocolate macaroon / **Pillsbury**	168	30–40
Fudge nut crown / **Pillsbury**	144	30–40
Lemon blueberry / **Pillsbury**	132	30–40
Marble / **Pillsbury**	144	30–40
Pound / **Pillsbury**	144	30–40
Triple fudge / **Pillsbury**	156	30–40
Butter / **Duncan Hines**	156	40–50
Butter / **Pillsbury Plus**	120	40–50
Butter Brickle / **Betty Crocker**	144	40–50
Butter fudge / **Duncan Hines**	156	40–50
Butter pecan / **Betty Crocker**	156	40–50
Cheesecake / **Pillsbury** No Bake	400	90–100
Cheesecake / **Jell-O**	88	40–50
Cheesecake / **Royal**	24	10–20

	FAT GRAMS	PERCENT OF CALORIES FROM FAT
Cherry / **Duncan Hines**	60	20–30
Cherry chip / **Betty Crocker**	60	20–30
Chocolate / **Betty Crocker** Pudding Cake	30	10–20
Chocolate / **Duncan Hines**	72	20–30
Chocolate almond / **Betty Crocker** Snackin' Cake	72	30–40
Chocolate chip / **Betty Crocker** Snackin' Cake	72	30–40
Chocolate chip / **Duncan Hines**	54	20–30
Chocolate chip, double / **Duncan Hines**	45	20–30
Chocolate, dark / **Pillsbury Plus**	144	40–50
Chocolate fudge / **Betty Crocker** Snackin' Cake	72	30–40
Chocolate fudge / **Betty Crocker**	168	40–50
Chocolate, German / **Betty Crocker**	156	40–50
Chocolate, German / **Pillsbury**	144	40–50
Chocolate, milk / **Betty Crocker**	144	40–50
Chocolate, sour cream / **Betty Crocker**	168	40–50
Chocolate, sour cream / **Duncan Hines**	72	20–30
Chocolate, Swiss / **Duncan Hines**	72	20–30
Chocolate w chocolate frosting / **Betty Crocker** Stir n' Frost	66	30–40
Coconut pecan / **Betty Crocker** Snackin' Cake	81	30–40
Cupcakes / **Flako**	5	30–40
Date nut / **Betty Crocker** Snackin' Cake	72	30–40
Devil's food / **Betty Crocker**	156	40–50
Devil's food / **Duncan Hines**	72	20–30
Devil's food / **Pillsbury**	144	40–50
Fudge marble / **Duncan Hines**	60	20–30
Fudge marble / **Pillsbury**	144	40–50

	FAT GRAMS	PERCENT OF CALORIES FROM FAT
Gingerbread / **Betty Crocker**	54	20–30
Gingerbread: 3-in sq / **Pillsbury**	4	10–20
Lemon / **Betty Crocker**		
Pudding Cake	30	40–50
Lemon w lemon frosting /		
Betty Crocker Stir n' Frost	48	30–40
Lemon / **Betty Crocker**	156	40–50
Lemon / **Duncan Hines**	60	20–30
Lemon / **Pillsbury Plus**	144	40–50
Lemon chiffon / **Betty Crocker**	48	10–20
Marble / **Betty Crocker**	156	40–50
Orange / **Betty Crocker**	156	40–50
Orange / **Duncan Hines**	60	20–30
Pineapple / **Duncan Hines**	60	20–30
Pineapple upside-down w topping /		
Betty Crocker	90	30–40
Pound / **Betty Crocker**	96	30–40
Spice / **Betty Crocker**	168	40–50
Spice / **Duncan Hines**	60	20–30
Spice w vanilla frosting /		
Betty Crocker Stir n' Frost	48	20–30
Spice raisin / **Betty Crocker**		
Snackin' Cake	54	20–30
Strawberry / **Betty Crocker**	156	40–50
Strawberry / **Duncan Hines**	60	20–30
Strawberry / **Pillsbury**	144	40–50
Struesel cake		
Cinnamon / **Pillsbury**	168	30–40
Devil's food / **Pillsbury**	156	30–40
Fudge marble / **Pillsbury**	168	30–40
German chocolate / **Pillsbury**	156	30–40
Lemon / **Pillsbury**	180	30–40
White / **Betty Crocker**	72	20–30
White / **Duncan Hines**	60	20–30
White / **Pillsbury**	120	30–40
White, sour cream / **Betty Crocker**	72	20–30

	FAT GRAMS	PERCENT OF CALORIES FROM FAT
Yellow / **Betty Crocker**	156	40–50
Yellow / **Betty Crocker**		
Butter Recipe	120	30–40
Yellow / **Duncan Hines**	60	20–30
Yellow w chocolate frosting /		
Betty Crocker Stir n' Frost	48	30–40
Yellow / **Pillsbury**	144	40–50

COFFEE CAKES

1 whole cake

Apple cinnamon mix, prepared /		
Pillsbury	56	20–30
Butter pecan, mix, prepared /		
Pillsbury	120	30–40
Cinnamon streusel, mix, prepared /		
Pillsbury	64	20–30
Coffee cake, mix prepared / **Aunt**		
Jemima Easy Mix	40	20–30
Sour cream, mix, prepared /		
Pillsbury	96	40–50

SNACK CAKES

Big Wheels: 1 cake / **Hostess**	10	50–60
Brownie, large: 1 brownie /		
Hostess	10	30–40
Brownie, small: 1 brownie /		
Hostess	6	30–40
Choco-Diles: 1 cake / **Hostess**	11	40–50
Creamies, chocolate: 1 pkg /		
Tastykake	10	30–40
Creamies, spice: 1 pkg / **Tastykake**	10	30–40
Crumb cake: 1 cake / **Hostess**	4	20–30
Cupcakes		
Buttercream filled: 1 pkg /		
Tastykake	8	30–40

	FAT GRAMS	PERCENT OF CALORIES FROM FAT
Chocolate: 1 cake /Hostess	5	20–30
Chocolate: 1 pkg / Tastykake	5	20–30
Chocolate, cream filled: 1 pkg / Tastykake	9	30–40
Orange: 1 cake /Hostess	4	20–30
Ding Dongs: 1 cake / Hostess	10	50–60
Donuts: 1 donut		
Hostess, plain	7	50–60
Hostess Crunch	4	30–40
Hostess Enrobed	9	60–70
Cinnamon / Hostess	6	40–50
Powdered / Hostess	6	40–50
Ho Ho's: 1 cake / Hostess	6	40–50
Juniors, chocolate: 1 pkg / Tastykake	12.2	30–40
Juniors, coconut: 1 pkg / Tastykake	11	30–40
Juniors, koffee kake: 1 pkg / Tastykake	15	40–50
Juniors, lemon: 1 pkg / Tastykake	7	20–30
Koffee Kake, cream filled: 1 pkg / Tastykake	12	40–50
Krimpets, butterscotch: 1 pkg / Tastykake	5.5	20–30
Krimpets, jelly: 1 pkg / Tastykake	3.5	10–20
Krimpies, chocolate: 1 pkg / Tastykake	9	30–40
Krimpies, vanilla: 1 pkg / Tastykake	8	30–40
Macaroon, fudge: 1 cake / Hostess	9	30–40
Oatmeal cake, creme filled: 2 oz / Frito-Lay	11.3	30–40
Oatmeal raisin: 1 pkg / Tastykake Bars	10	30–40
Orange treats: 1 pkg / Tastykake	7	20–30
Sno Balls: 1 cake / Hostess	4	20–30
Suzy Q: 1 cake / Hostess	9	30–40
Suzy Q, chocolate: 1 cake / Hostess	9	30–40
Tandy Takes, peanut butter: 1 pkg / Tastykake	11	50–60

	FAT GRAMS	PERCENT OF CALORIES FROM FAT
Tandy Takes, chocolate: 1 pkg / **Tastykake**	9.5	40–50
Tasty Klairs, chocolate: 1 pkg / **Tastykake**	24	40–50
Teens, chocolate: 1 pkg / **Tastykake**	6	20–30
Tempty, chocolate cream: 1 pkg / **Tastykake**	4	10–20
Tempty, lemon: 1 pkg / **Tastykake**	8	20–30
Tiger Tails: 1 cake / **Hostess**	13	20–30
Twinkies: 1 cake / **Hostess**	4	20–30
Twinkies, devil's food: 1 cake / **Hostess**	5	30–40

Candy

	FAT GRAMS	PERCENT OF CALORIES FROM FAT
Chocolate and chocolate-covered bars: 1 oz unless noted		
Hershey's	10	50–60
w almonds / **Hershey's**	10	50–60
Nestlé's	8	40–50
w almonds / **Nestlé's**	9	50–60
Baby Ruth: 1 bar	11	30–40
Butterfinger: 1 bar	10	40–50
Choco'Lite / **Nestlé's**	8	40–50
Choc-O-Roon / **Frito-Lay**	7.6	20–30
Crunch / **Nestlé's**	8	40–50

	FAT GRAMS	PERCENT OF CALORIES FROM FAT
Kit Kat: 1.1 oz / **Hershey's**	8	40–50
Krackel / **Hershey's**	9	40–50
Mr. Goodbar: 1.3 oz	13	50–60
$100,000 / **Nestlé's**	6	30–40
Rally: 1.5 oz / **Hershey's**	11	40–50
Reggie: 1 bar	17	50–60
Special Dark Bar: 1.2 oz / **Hershey's**	10	50–60
Chocolate and chocolate covered bits		
Hershey-ets: 1.1 oz	6	30–40
Kisses: 1 oz / **Hershey's**	9	50–60
Rolo: 1 piece / **Hershey's**	1.2	30–40
Chocolate Parfait: 1¾ oz / **Pearson**	8	30–40
Coffioca: 1¾ oz / **Pearson**	8	30–40
Coffee Nip: 1¾ oz / **Pearson**	5	20–30
Licorice Nip: 1¾ oz / **Pearson**	5	20–30
Mint Parfait: 1¾ oz / **Pearson**	8	30–40
Peanut candy, canned: 1 oz / **Planters** Old Fashioned	9	50–60
Peanut butter bar: 1¾ oz / **Frito-Lay**	16.8	50–60
Peanut Butter Cup: 1 piece / **Reese's**	5.5	50–60

DIETETIC CANDY

	FAT GRAMS	PERCENT OF CALORIES FROM FAT
Chocolate bars		
Almond: ¾ oz bar / **Estee**	8.1	60–70
Almond: 3 oz bar, 1 section / **Estee**	2.7	60–70
Bittersweet: 3 oz bar, 1 section / **Estee**	2.8	60–70
Crunch: ⅝ oz bar / **Estee**	6.2	60–70
Crunch: 2½ oz bar, 1 section / **Estee**	2.1	60–70
Fruit and nut: 3 oz pkg, 1 section / **Estee**	2.5	60–70
Milk: 3 oz pkg, 1 section / **Estee**	2.6	60–70
Milk: ¾ oz bar / **Estee**	7.8	60–70

	GRAMS FAT	PERCENT OF FROM FAT CALORIES
Chocolates, boxed: 1 piece		
Peanut butter cups / Estee	3.2	60–70
Raisins, chocolate-covered / Estee	.3	40–50
T.V. Mix / Estee	.6	60–70
Estee-Ets, plain	.4	60–70
Estee-Ets, peanut	.5	60–70
Gum drops, fruit / Estee	0	0
Gum drops, licorice / Estee	0	0
Hard candies, assorted / Estee	0	0
Hard candies, cough / Estee	0	0
Hard candies, creme / Estee	0	0
Hard candies, peppermint / Estee	0	0
Mint candies, assorted / Estee 5 Pak	0	0
Mint candies, assorted fruit / Estee 5 Pak	0	0
Mint candies, peppermint / Estee	0	0
Mint candies, sour cherry / Estee	0	0
Mint candies, sour lemon / Estee	0	0
Mint candies, sour orange / Estee	0	0
Mint candies, spearmint / Estee	0	0

Cereals

DRY READY-TO-SERVE

Measurements vary according to what companies consider appropriate one-serving sizes. The servings generally are one ounce in weight.

	FAT GRAMS	PERCENT OF CALORIES FROM FAT
All-Bran: ⅓ cup / **Kellogg's**	1	10–20
Alpha-Bits: 1 cup / **Post**	1	0–10
Apple Jacks: 1 cup / **Kellogg's**	0	0–10
Boo Berry: 1 cup / **General Mills**	1	0–10
Bran, plain, added sugar, defatted wheat germ: 1 cup	1.4	0–10
Bran, plain, added sugar, malt extract: 1 cup	1.4	0–10
Bran Buds: ⅓ cup / **Kellogg's**	0	0–10
Bran Chex: ⅔ cup / **Ralston Purina**	.9	0–10
Bran Flakes 40%: ⅔ cup / **Kellogg's**	1	0–10
Bran Flakes 40%: ⅔ cup / **Post**	1	0–10
Buck Wheats: ¾ cup / **General Mills**	1	0–10
C.W. Post: ½ cup	5	30–40
C.W. Post w raisins: ½ cup	5	30–40
Cap'n Crunch: ¾ cup	2.6	10–20
Cap'n Crunch's Crunchberries: ¾ cup	2.6	10–20
Cap'n Crunch's Peanut Butter: ¾ cup	3.8	20–30
Cheerios: 1¼ cup / **General Mills**	2	10–20
Chocolate Crazy Cow: 1 cup / **General Mills**	1	0–10
Cocoa Krispies: ¾ cup / **Kellogg's**	0	0–10
Cocoa Pebbles: ⅞ cup / **Post**	2	10–20
Cocoa Puffs: 1 cup / **General Mills**	1	0–10
Concentrate: ⅓ cup / **Kellogg's**	0	0–10

	FAT GRAMS	PERCENT OF CALORIES FROM FAT
Cookie Crisp, chocolate chip: 1 cup / **Ralston Purina**	1	0–10
Cookie Crisp, vanilla wafer: 1 cup / **Ralston Purina**	1	0–10
Corn Chex: 1 cup / **Ralston Purina**	.1	0–10
Corn flakes: 1 cup / **General Mills** Country	1	0–10
Corn flakcs: 1 cup / **Kellogg's**	0	0–10
Corn flakes: 1¼ cup / **Post** Toasties	0	0–10
Corn flakes: 1 cup / **Ralston Purina**	.1	0–10
Corn flakes: 1 cup / **Safeway**	1	0–10
Corn flakes, sugar-coated: ⅔ cup / **Kellogg's** Frosted	0	0–10
Corn Total: 1 cup / **General Mills**	1	0–10
Corny-Snaps: 1 cup / **Kellogg's**	2	10–20
Count Chocula: 1 cup / **General Mills**	1	0–10
Country Morning: ⅓ cup / **Kellogg's**	5	30–40
Country Morning w raisins and dates: ⅓ cup / **Kellogg's**	5	30–40
Cracklin' Bran: ⅓ cup / **Kellogg's**	4	30–40
Crispy Rice: 1 cup / **Ralston Purina**	.2	0–10
Franken Berry: 1 cup / **General Mills**	1	0–10
Froot Loops: 1 cup / **Kellogg's**	1	0–10
Frosty O's: 1 cup / **General Mills**	1	0–10
Fruit Brute: 1 cup / **General Mills**	1	0–10
Fruity Pebbles: ⅞ cup / **Post**	2	10–20
Golden Grahams: 1 cup / **General Mills**	1	0–10
Granola: 1 oz / **Nature Valley**	5	30–40
Granola w cinnamon and raisins: 1 oz / **Nature Valley**	5	30–40
Granola w coconut and honey: 1 oz / **Nature Valley**	5	30–40
Granola w fruit and nuts: 1 oz / **Nature Valley**	4	20–30

	FAT GRAMS	PERCENT OF CALORIES FROM FAT
Grape-Nuts: ¼ cup / **Post**	0	0–10
Grape-Nut Flakes: ⅞ cup / **Post**	0	0–10
Heartland, plain: ¼ cup	4	30–40
Heartland, coconut: ¼ cup	5	30–40
Heartland, raisin: ¼ cup	4	30–40
Honeycomb: 1⅓ cup / **Post**	1	0–10
Kaboom: 1 cup / **General Mills**	1	0–10
King Vitamin: ¾ cup	2.4	10–20
Kix: 1½ cup / **General Mills**	1	0–10
Life: ⅔ cup	.5	0–5
Lucky Charms: 1 cup / **General Mills**	1	0–10
Mini-Wheats: about 5 biscuits / **Kellogg's**	0	0–10
Mini-Wheats, frosted: about 4 biscuits / **Kellogg's**	0	0–10
Oat flakes, fortified: ⅔ cup / **Post**	1	0–10
Pep: ¾ cup / **Kellogg's**	0	0–10
Product 19: ¾ cup / **Kellogg's**	0	0–10
Quaker 100% Natural: ¼ cup	6.3	40–50
Quaker 100% Natural w apples and cinnamon: ¼ cup	5.5	30–40
Quaker 100% Natural w raisins and dates: ¼ cup	5.6	30–40
Quisp: 1 1/6 cup	2.6	10–20
Raisin bran: ¾ cup / **Kellogg's**	1	0–10
Raisin bran: ½ cup / **Post**	1	0–10
Raisin bran: ½ cup / **Ralston Purina**	.2	0–10
Raisin bran: ½ cup / **Safeway**	1	0–10
Rice: 1 cup / **Safeway** Crispy Rice	0	0–10
Rice, frosted: 1 cup / **Kellogg's**	0	0–10
Rice, puffed: ½ oz / **Malt-O-Meal**	0	0–10
Rice, puffed: 1 cup / **Quaker**	.1	0–10
Rice Chex: 1⅛ cup / **Ralston Purina**	.5	0–10
Rice Krinkles, frosted: ⅞ cup / **Post**	0	0–10
Rice Krispies: 1 cup / **Kellogg's**	0	0–10
Special K: 1¼ cup / **Kellogg's**	0	0–10

	FAT GRAMS	PERCENT OF CALORIES FROM FAT
Strawberry Crazy Cow: 1 cup / **General Mills**	1	0–10
Sugar Corn Pops: 1 cup / **Kellogg's**	0	0–10
Sugar Frosted Flakes: ¾ cup / **Ralston Purina**	.3	0–10
Sugar Smacks: ¾ cup / **Kellogg's**	0	0–10
Super Sugar Crisp: ⅞ cup / **Post**	1	0–10
Tastecos: 1¼ cup / **Safeway**	1	0–10
Toasty-O's: 1 oz	2	10–20
Total: 1 cup / **General Mills**	1	0–10
Trix: 1 cup / **General Mills**	1	0–10
Wheat, puffed: ½ oz / **Malt-O-Meal**	0	0–10
Wheat, puffed: 1 cup / **Quaker**	.2	0–10
Wheat, shredded: 1 biscuit / **Quaker**	.2	0–10
Wheat Chex: ⅔ cup / **Ralston Purina**	.9	0–10
Wheaties: 1 cup / **General Mills**	1	0–10

TO BE COOKED

Measurements vary

	FAT GRAMS	PERCENT OF CALORIES FROM FAT
Barley, pearled: ¼ cup uncooked (1 cup cooked) / **Quaker** Scotch Brand	.5	0–10
Barley, pearled: ¼ cup uncooked (¾ cup cooked) / **Quaker** Scotch Brand Quick	.5	0–10
Farina: 1 cup cooked / **H-O** Cream Enriched	0	0–10
Farina: ⅔ cup / **Pillsbury**	0	0–10
Farina: ⅔ cup, prepared w milk and salt / **Pillsbury**	7	30–40
Farina: 1/6 cup uncooked / **Quaker** Hot 'n Creamy	.2	0–10
Grits: ¼ cup uncooked / **Albers**	0	0–10
Grits: 1/6 cup uncooked / **3-Minute Brand** Quick	1	0–10

	FAT GRAMS	PERCENT OF CALORIES FROM FAT
Grits: 1 packet / **Quaker** Instant Grits Product	.1	0–10
Grits, hominy, white: 3 tbsp / **Aunt Jemima** Quick Enriched	.2	0–10
Grits, hominy, white: 3 tbsp /**Aunt Jemima** Regular	.2	0–10
Grits, hominy, white: 3 tbsp / **Quaker** Regular	.2	0–10
Grits, hominy, white: 3 tbsp / **Quaker** Quick	.2	0–10
Grits w artificial cheese flavor: 1 packet / **Quaker** Instant Grits Product	1	0–10
Grits w imitation bacon bits: 1 packet / **Quaker** Instant Grits Product	.4	0–10
Grits w imitation ham bits: 1 packet / **Quaker** Instant Grits Product	.3	0–10
Malt-O-Meal Chocolate: 1 oz uncooked (about ¾ cup cooked)	0	0–10
Malt-O-Meal Quick: 1 oz uncooked (about ¾ cup cooked)	0	0–10
Oats and oatmeal		
H-O Old Fashioned: ¾ cup cooked	2	10–20
H-O Quick: ¾ cup cooked	2	10–20
Harvest Quick: 1 oz uncooked	2	10–20
Quaker Quick: ⅓ cup uncooked	1.9	10–20
Quaker Old Fashioned: ⅓ cup uncooked	1.9	10–20
Ralston Purina: 1 oz uncooked	1.8	10–20
Ralston Purina Quick: 1 oz uncooked	1.8	10–20
3-Minute Brand Quick: 1 oz uncooked	2	10–20
Safeway Quick: ⅓ cup uncooked	2.5	10–20
Instant: ½ cup uncooked / **H-O**	2	10–20

	FAT GRAMS	PERCENT OF CALORIES FROM FAT
Instant: 1 packet / **H-O**	1.7	10–20
Instant: 1 packet / **H-O** Sweet and Mellow	1.7	10–20
Instant: 1 packet / **Quaker** Regular	1.7	10–20
Instant: 1 packet / **3-Minute Brand** Stir n' Eat	2	10–20
Instant w apple and brown sugar: 1 packet / **3-Minute Brand** Stir n' Eat	2	10–20
Instant w apples and cinnamon: 1 packet / **Quaker**	1.6	10–20
Instant w bran and raisins: 1 packet / **Quaker**	1.7	10–20
Instant w cinnamon and spice: 1 packet / **Quaker**	1.8	0–10
Instant w maple and brown sugar: 1 packet / **H-O**	1.8	0–10
Instant w maple and brown sugar: 1 packet / **Quaker**	1.9	10–20
Instant w raisins and spice: 1 packet / **H-O**	1.6	0–10
Instant w raisins and spice: 1 packet / **Quaker**	1.8	10–20
Ralston: 1 oz (uncooked) / **Ralston Purina**	.3	0–10
Ralston: 1 oz (uncooked) / **Ralston Purina** Instant	.3	0–10
Whole Wheat: ⅓ cup uncooked (⅔ cup cooked) / **Quaker** Pettijohns	.5	0–10

Cheese

NATURAL CHEESE

1 oz unless noted	FAT GRAMS	PERCENT OF CALORIES FROM FAT
Blue	8.1	70–80
Brick	8.4	70–80
Brie	7.8	70–80
Camembert	6.9	70–80
Caraway	8.3	70–80
Cheddar	9.4	70–80
Cheshire	8.7	70–80
Colby	9.1	70–80
Edam	7.8	70–80
Farmer	2.8	50–60
Feta	6.0	70–80
Fontina	8.8	70–80
Gjetost	8.4	50–60
Gouda	7.8	70–80
Gruyere	9.2	70–80
Limburger	7.7	70–80
Monterey	8.6	70–80
Mozzarella	6.1	60–70
Mozzarella, low moisture	7	60–70
Mozzarella, part skim	4.5	50–60
Mozzarella, low moisture, part skim	4.8	50–60
Muenster	8.5	70–80
Neufchâtel	6.6	70–80
Parmesan, grated	8.5	60–70
Parmesan, hard	7.3	60–70
Port du Salut	8	70–80
Provolone	7.5	60–70
Ricotta, whole milk: 1 cup	31.9	60–70

	FAT GRAMS	PERCENT OF CALORIES FROM FAT
Ricotta, partially skim milk: 1 cup	19.4	50–60
Romano	7.6	60–70
Roquefort	8.7	70–80
Swiss	7.8	60–70
Tilsit	7.4	60–70

PASTEURIZED PROCESS CHEESES

1 oz

American	8.9	70–80
Pimento	8.9	70–80
Swiss	7	60–70

COTTAGE CHEESE

Creamed		
Friendship: 4 oz	5	30–40
Lucerne: ½ cup	5	30–40
Meadow Gold: ½ cup	5	30–40
w chives: ½ cup / **Lucerne**	5	30–40
w fruit salad: 4 oz / **Friendship**		
Caloric Meter	2	10–20
w fruit salad: ½ cup / **Lucerne**	5	20–30
w pineapple: 4 oz / **Friendship**	4	20–30
w pineapple: ½ cup / **Lucerne**	5	20–30
w vegetable salad: 4 oz / **Friendship**		
Garden Salad	5	30–40
Dry, pot style: ½ cup / **Breakstone**	1	0–10
Dry: ½ cup / **Lucerne**	1	0–10
Low fat		
Breakstone: ½ cup	2	10–20
Breakstone skim milk, large curd:		
½ cup	1	10–20
Friendship Calorie Meter: 4 oz	2	10–20
Friendship Pot Style: 4 oz	2	10–20
Lite-Line: ½ cup	1	0–10
Lucerne Low fat: ½ cup	2	10–20

	FAT GRAMS	PERCENT OF CALORIES FROM FAT
Viva Low Fat	2	10–20
Weight Watchers Lowfat: ½ cup	1	0–10

CREAM CHEESE

	FAT GRAMS	PERCENT OF CALORIES FROM FAT
Philadelphia Brand: 1 oz	10	90–100
Lucerne: 1 oz	10	90–100
Imitation: 1 oz / **Philadelphia Brand**	4	70–80

CHEESE FOOD

	FAT GRAMS	PERCENT OF CALORIES FROM FAT
American: 1 slice / **Lucerne**	4.7	60–70
American: 1 slice / **Safeway**	9	80–90
American: 1 oz / **Swift Pauly**	7	60–70
Blue: 1 oz / **Wispride** Cold Pack	7	60–70
Cheddar flavor: 1 oz / **Wispride** Cold Pack	7	60–70
Pimento: 1 oz / **Swift Pauly**	7	60–70
Sweet Munchee: 1 oz / **Swift Pauly**	8	70–80
Swiss: 1 oz / **Swift Pauly**	7	60–70
Swiss: 1 oz / **Wispride** Cold Pack	7	60–70

CHEESE SPREADS

	FAT GRAMS	PERCENT OF CALORIES FROM FAT
Cheddar flavor, processed: 1 oz / **Wispride**	6	60–70
Velveeta, processed: 1 oz / **Kraft**	6	60–70

WELSH RAREBIT

	FAT GRAMS	PERCENT OF CALORIES FROM FAT
Frozen: 5 oz / **Green Giant** Boil-In-Bag Toast Toppers	15	60–70

Chewing Gum

No fat

Chinese Foods

	FAT GRAMS	PERCENT OF CALORIES FROM FAT
Apple-cinnamon roll, frozen: 1 roll / **La Choy**	.8	10–20
Bamboo shoots, canned: 8½ oz can / **Chun King**	.3	0–10
Bean sprouts, canned: 16 oz can / **Chun King**	.4	0–10
Bean sprouts, canned: 1 cup / **La Choy**	.1	0–10
Chop suey, beef, frozen: 32 oz / **Banquet** Buffet Supper	11.8	20–30
Chop suey, beef, frozen: 7 oz / **Banquet** Cookin' Bag	1.4	10–20
Chop suey, vegetables, canned: 1 cup / **La Choy**	.2	0–10
Chow mein, canned		
Beef: 1 cup / **La Choy**	2.3	20–30
Beef: 1 cup / **La Choy** Bi-Pack	1.1	10–20
Chicken: 1 cup / **La Choy**	2.3	30–40
Chicken: 1 cup / **La Choy** Bi-Pack	3.4	30–40
Chicken: 1 cup / **La Choy** 50 oz	3.6	30–40
Meatless: 1 cup / **La Choy**	1.4	20–30

	FAT GRAMS	PERCENT OF CALORIES FROM FAT
Meatless: 1 cup / **La Choy** 50 oz	.2	20–30
Mushroom: 1 cup / **La Choy** Bi-Pack	3.4	30–40
Pepper oriental: 1 cup / **La Choy**	1.4	10–20
Pepper oriental: 1 cup / **La Choy** Bi-Pack	1	10–20
Pork: 7½ oz / **Hormel Short Orders**	7	40–50
Pork: 1 cup / **La Choy** Bi-Pack	6	40–50
Shrimp: 1 cup / **La Choy**	1.6	20–30
Shrimp: 1 cup / **La Choy** Bi-Pack	5.8	40–50
Vegetables: 16 oz can / **Chun King**	.4	0–10
Chow mein, frozen		
Beef: **La Choy**	2	10–20
Chicken: 32 oz / **Banquet** Buffet Supper	6.4	10–20
Chicken: 7 oz / **Banquet** Cookin' Bag	1.6	10–20
Chicken: 1 cup / **La Choy**	4	30–40
Chicken wo noodles: 9 oz / **Green Giant** Boil-in-Bag	2	10–20
Shrimp: 1 cup / **La Choy**	.7	0–10
Egg rolls, chicken, frozen: 1 roll / **La Choy**	1.2	30–40
Egg rolls, lobster, frozen: 1 roll / **La Choy**	.9	30–40
Fried rice, chicken, canned: 1 cup / **La Choy**	3.8	0–10
Fried rice, Chinese style, canned: 1 cup / **La Choy**	3.8	0–10
Fried rice and pork, frozen: 1 cup / **La Choy**	6	20–30
Noodles, chow mein, canned: 1 cup / **La Choy**	17.6	50–60
Noodles, ramen-beef, canned: 1 cup / **La Choy**	7.5	30–40

	FAT GRAMS	PERCENT OF CALORIES FROM FAT
Noodles, ramen-chicken, canned:		
1 cup / **La Choy**	6.8	30–40
Noodles, ramen-oriental, canned:		
1 cup / **La Choy**	8.6	30–40
Noodles, rice, canned: 1 cup /		
La Choy	9.2	30–40
Noodles, wide chow mein, canned:		
1 cup / **La Choy**	16.6	50–60
Pea pods, frozen: 1 pkg / **La Choy**	.3	0–10
Pepper oriental, frozen: 1 cup /		
La Choy	2	10–20
Sweet & sour pork, frozen:		
1 cup / **La Choy**	3	10–20
Vegetables, mixed Chinese, canned:		
1 cup / **La Choy**	.2	0–10
Water chestnuts, canned:		
8½ oz / **Chun King**	.3	0–10
Won Ton, frozen: 1 cup / **La Choy**	2	10/20

Chips, Crisps
and Similar Snacks

	FAT GRAMS	PERCENT OF CALORIES FROM FAT
1 oz unless noted		
Cheddar Bitz / Frito-Lay	4.7	30–40
Cheeze Balls / **Planters**	10	50–60

	FAT GRAMS	PERCENT OF CALORIES FROM FAT
Cheez Curls / **Planters**	10	50–60
Chee.Tos / **Frito-Lay**	10.3	50–60
Corn chips		
Fritos	10.2	50–60
Planters	11	50–60
Barbecue-flavored / **Fritos**	9.7	50–60
Corn Nuggets, toasted: 1⅜ oz /		
Frito-Lay	5.4	20–30
Funyuns	6	30–40
Munchos / **Frito-Lay**	10	50–60
Potato chips		
Frito-Lay	10.7	60–70
Frito-Lay Natural Style	10	60–70
Frito-Lay Ruffles	9.4	60–70
Planters Stackable	8	40–50
Pringle's	10	60–70
Pringle's Country Style	11	60–70
Pringle's Extra Rippled	10	60–70
Barbecue-flavored: **Lay's**	10.2	50–60
Sour cream-and-onion-flavored / **Lay's**	9.8	50–60
Potato sticks, canned: 1½ oz / **O & C**	15	50–60
Puffs-Crunchy, cheese-flavored / **Chee.Tos**	9.6	50–60
Pumpkin and squash seed kernels, dry, hulled: 1 cup	65.4	70–80
Rinds, fried, pork / **Baken-Ets**	7.5	40–50
Snack Sticks, lightly salted / **Pepperidge Farm**	4	30–40
Snack Sticks, pumpernickel / **Pepperidge Farm**	4	30–40
Snack Sticks, sesame / **Pepperidge Farm**	5	30–40
Snack Sticks, whole wheat / **Pepperidge Farm**	4	30–40

	FAT GRAMS	PERCENT OF CALORIES FROM FAT
Sesame seeds, dry, hulled, decorticated:		
1 tbsp	4.3	80–90
Sunflower seeds, in hull: 1 cup	21.7	70–80
Tortilla chips / **Doritos**	6.4	40–50
Tortilla chips / **Planters** Nacho	7	40–50
Tortilla chips / **Planters** Taco	7	40–50
Tortilla chips, nacho cheese flavor /		
Doritos	6.9	40–50
Tortilla chips, taco flavor / **Doritos**	6.7	40–50
Wheat chips, imitation bacon-flavored /		
Bakon-Snacks	9.1	50–60

Chocolate and Chips

	FAT GRAMS	PERCENT OF CALORIES FROM FAT
For Baking: 1 oz unless noted		
Chips		
Butterscotch-flavored / **Nestlé's**		
Morsels	7	40–50
Chocolate: ¼ cup / **Hershey's**	14	50–60
Chocolate / **Nestlé's** Morsels	9	50–60
Chocolate, flavor / **Baker's**	7	40–50
Chocolate, semi-sweet: 1.5 oz /		
Hershey's	12	40–50
Chocolate, semi-sweet: 1.5 oz /		
Hershey's Mini	12	40–50
Chocolate, semi-sweet / **Nestlé's**		
Morsels	8	40–50

	FAT GRAMS	PERCENT OF CALORIES FROM FAT
Peanut butter-flavored / **Reese's**	8	40–50
Choco-bake / **Nestlé's**	14	70–80
Chocolate, solid / **Hershey's**	16	70–80
Chocolate, solid, German's swt / **Baker's**	9	50–60
Chocolate, solid, semi-swt / **Baker's**	9	60–70
Chocolate, unswt / **Baker's**	14	90–100

Cocktail Mixes

No fat

Cocoa

	FAT GRAMS	PERCENT OF CALORIES FROM FAT
Cocoa: 1 oz / **Hershey's**	4	30–40
Cocoa: 1 tbsp / **Marvel**	1	30–40
Cocoa, chocolate flavor: ¾ oz / **Nestlé's**	1	10–20
Cocoa, mix: 1 oz / **Hershey's**	2	10–20
Cocoa, mix: 3 tbsp / **Hershey's** Instant	1	10–20
prepared w 8 oz milk / **Hershey's** Instant	10	30–40

	FAT GRAMS	PERCENT OF CALORIES FROM FAT
Cocoa, mix: 1 oz / **Nestlé's**	1	0–10
Cocoa, mix: 1 oz / **Ovaltine**	3	20–30
Cocoa, mix: .69 oz / **Ovaltine** Reduced Calorie	2	20–30
Cocoa mix, all flavors, instant: 1 oz / **Carnation**	1.2	0–10

Coconut

	FAT GRAMS	PERCENT OF CALORIES FROM FAT
Meat, fresh, in shell: 1 coconut	140	90–100
Meat: 1 piece (2 x 2 x ½ in)	15.9	90–100
Meat, shredded or grated: 1 cup	28.2	90–100
Plain: ¼ cup / **Baker's** Angel Flake	6	60–70
Plain: ¼ cup / **Baker's** Premium Shred	7	60–70
Plain: ¼ cup / **Baker's** Southern Style	7	60–70
Plain, shredded: ¼ cup / **Durkee**	7	60–70
Cookie-coconut: ¼ cup / **Baker's**	9	50–60

Coffee

No fat

Condiments

	FAT GRAMS	PERCENT OF CALORIES FROM FAT
A.1 Sauce / 1 tbsp	0	0–10
Catsup: 1 tbsp / **Del Monte**	0	0–10
Catsup: 1 tbsp / **Tillie Lewis**	0	0–10
Hot sauce: 1 tsp / **Frank's**	.4	0–10
Mustard, prepared		
Brown: 1 tbsp / **French's** Brown 'n Spicy	1	60–70
Brown: 1 tsp / **Mr. Mustard**	.8	60–70
Cream salad: 1 tbsp / **French's**	1	90–100
Dijon: 1 tsp / **Grey Poupon**	.4	70–80
w horseradish: 1 tbsp / **French's**	1	60–70
w onion: 1 tbsp / **French's**	1	30–40
Yellow: 1 tbsp / **French's** Medford	1	50–60
Seafood, cocktail: ¼ cup / **Del Monte**	1	10–20
Seafood, cocktail: 1 oz / **Pfeiffer**	2.5	20–30
Soy sauce: 1 tbsp / **La Choy**	.1	0–10
Steak sauce: 1 tbsp / **Steak Supreme**	.1	0–10
Taco sauce: 1 tbsp / **Ortego**	.1	0–10
Tartar sauce: 1 tbsp / **Best Foods**	7.9	90–100
Tartar sauce: 1 tbsp / **Hellman's**	7.9	90–100
Tartar sauce: 1 tbsp / **Seven Seas**	9	90–100
Vinegar: 1 fl oz / **Regina**	0	0
Worcestershire: 1 tbsp / **French's**	0	0

---

*Although some condiments, like mustard, derive a high percent of this caloric fat, you usually do not eat enough to consume many fat grams.

Cookies

	FAT GRAMS	PERCENT OF CALORIES FROM FAT
1 piece as packaged unless noted		
Adelaide / **Pepperidge Farm**	2.7	40–50
Angel Puffs / **Stella D'Oro** Dietetic	1	40–50
Angelica Goodies / **Stella D'Oro**	3.9	30–40
Anginetti / **Stella D'Oro**	1.1	30–40
Animal crackers / **Sunshine**	.3	20–30
Animal crackers, iced / **Sunshine**	1.2	40–50
Animal crackers, Barnum's Animals / **Nabisco**	.3	20–30
Anisette sponge / **Stella D'Oro**	.6	10–20
Anisette toast / **Stella D'Oro**	.5	0–10
Apple pastry / **Stella D'Oro** Dietetic	3.8	30–40
Applesauce / **Sunshine**	3.8	30–40
Applesauce, iced / **Sunshine**	3.8	30–40
Arrowroot / **Sunshine**	.4	20–30
Assortment / **Stella D'Oro** Hostess with the Mostest	2.1	40–50
Assortment / **Stella D'Oro** Lady Stella	1.9	40–50
Aunt Sally, iced / **Sunshine**	1.6	10–20
Big Treat / **Sunshine**	5	20–30
Biscos / **Nabisco**	2	40–50
Bordeaux / **Pepperidge Farm**	1.6	30–40
Breakfast Treats / **Stella D'Oro**	3.9	30–40
Brown Sugar / **Pepperidge Farm**	2.3	40–50
Brussels / **Pepperidge Farm**	3.3	50–60
Butter-flavored / **Nabisco**	.9	30–40
Butter-flavored / **Sunshine**	.9	30–40
Cameo creme sandwich / **Nabisco**	2.5	30–40
Capri / **Pepperidge Farm**	5	50–60
Chessman / **Pepperidge Farm**	2	40–50

	FAT GRAMS	PERCENT OF CALORIES FROM FAT
Chinese dessert cookies / **Stella D'Oro**	8.8	40–50
Chip-A-Roos / **Sunshine**	2.9	40–50
Chocolate brownie / **Pepperidge Farm**	3.7	50–60
Chocolate chip / **Estee** Dietetic	1	30–40
Chocolate chip / **Pepperidge Farm**	2	40–50
Chocolate chip coconut / **Sunshine**	4.3	40–50
Chocolate fudge sandwich / **Sunshine**	3.7	40–50
Chocolate-strawberry wafers, dietetic, single serving pkg: 1 pkg / **Estee**	4.6	40–50
Cinnamon sugar / **Pepperidge Farm**	2.3	30–40
Cinnamon toast / **Sunshine**	.3	20–30
Coconut Bar / **Sunshine**	2.3	40–50
Coconut cookies / **Stella D'Oro** Dietetic	2.4	40–50
Coconut macaroons / **Nabisco**	4	40–50
Como Delight / **Stella D'Oro**	7.1	40–50
Cream Lunch / **Sunshine**	1.4	20–30
Crescents, almond-flavored / **Nabisco**	1.3	30–40
Cup Custard, chocolate / **Sunshine**	3.3	10–20
Cup Custard, vanilla / **Sunshine**	3.3	10–20
Date-Nut Granola / **Pepperidge Farm**	2.7	40–50
Dixie Vanilla / **Sunshine**	1.8	20–30
Egg biscuits / **Stella D'Oro**	.9	10–20
Egg biscuits / **Stella D'Oro** Dietetic	1	10–20
Egg biscuits, anise / **Stella D'Oro** Roman	5.1	30–40
Egg biscuits, rum and brandy / **Stella D'Oro** Roman	5.1	30–40
Egg biscuits, sugared / **Stella D'Oro**	1.4	20–30
Egg biscuits, vanilla / **Stella D'Oro** Roman	5.1	30–40
Egg Jumbo / **Stella D'Oro**	.5	10–20
Fig bar: 2 oz / **Frito-Lay**	3.4	10–20
Fig bar / **Sunshine**	.8	10–20

	FAT GRAMS	PERCENT OF CALORIES FROM FAT
Fig pastry / **Stella D'Oro** Dietetic	3.8	30–40
Fudge chip / **Pepperidge Farm**	2.7	40–50
Ginger snap / **Nabisco**	.7	20–30
Ginger snap / **Sunshine**	.6	20–30
Gingerman / **Pepperidge Farm**	1.3	30–40
Golden bars / **Stella D'Oro**	4.8	30–40
Golden Fruit / **Sunshine**	.6	0–10
Graham crackers / **Nabisco** Honey Maid	.7	20–30
Graham crackers / **Sunshine** Sweet-Tooth	2.2	40–50
Hydrox / **Sunshine**	2.2	40–50
Hydrox, mint / **Sunshine**	2.2	40–50
Hydrox, vanilla / **Sunshine**	2.3	40–50
Irish oatmeal / **Pepperidge Farm**	2.3	40–50
Kichel / **Stella D'Oro** Dietetic	.5	50–60
Lady Joan, iced / **Sunshine**	1.9	40–50
Lady Joan / **Sunshine**	2.4	50–60
LaLanne Sesame / **Sunshine**	.7	40–50
LaLanne Soya / **Sunshine**	.9	40–50
Lemon / **Sunshine**	3.7	40–50
Lemon Coolers / **Sunshine**	1.1	30–40
Lemon nut crunch / **Pepperidge Farm**	3.3	40–50
Lemon Thins, dietetic / **Estee**	1	30–40
Lido / **Pepperidge Farm**	5.5	50–60
Love Cookies / **Stella D'Oro** Dietetic	5.3	40–50
Mallopuffs / **Sunshine**	1.6	20–30
Margherite, chocolate / **Stella D'Oro**	3.2	30–40
Margherite, vanilla / **Stella D'Oro**	3	30–40
Milano / **Pepperidge Farm**	3.7	50–60
Mint Milano / **Pepperidge Farm**	4	50–60
Molasses crisps / **Pepperidge Farm**	1.3	30–40
Molasses and spice / **Sunshine**	1.8	20–30
Nassau / **Pepperidge Farm**	4.5	50–60
'Nilla Wafers / **Nabisco**	.6	30–40

	FAT GRAMS	PERCENT OF CALORIES FROM FAT
Nutter Butter / **Nabisco**	3	30–40
Oatmeal		
Sunshine	2.3	30–40
Almond / **Pepperidge Farm**	2.7	40–50
Iced / **Sunshine**	2.2	20–30
Marmalade / **Pepperidge Farm**	2.7	40–50
Peanut butter / **Sunshine**	3.6	40–50
Raisin, dietetic / **Estee**	1	30–40
Raisin / **Nabisco**	3	30–40
Raisin / **Pepperidge Farm**	2.7	40–50
Orbit Creme Sandwich / **Sunshine**	2.4	40–50
Oreo / **Nabisco**	2	30–40
Orleans / **Pepperidge Farm**	2	50–60
Peach apricot pastry / **Stella D'Oro**	3.6	30–40
Peach apricot pastry / **Stella D'Oro**		
Dietetic	4	30–40
Peanut / **Pepperidge Farm**	2.3	40–50
Peanut butter wafers / **Sunshine**	1.4	30–40
Peanut creme patties / **Nabisco**	1.8	40–50
Pirouette / **Pepperidge Farm**	2.3	50–60
Pirouette, chocolate-laced /		
Pepperidge Farm	2.3	50–60
Prune pastry / **Stella D'Oro** Dietetic	3.9	30–40
Pfeffernusse / **Stella D'Oro**		
Spice Drops	.8	10–20
Raisin Bran / **Pepperidge Farm**	2.3	30–40
Raisin fruit biscuit / **Nabisco**	.6	0–10
Royal Nuggets / **Stella D'Oro** Dietetic	.1	80–90
St. Moritz / **Pepperidge Farm**	2.7	50–60
Sandwich		
Estee Dietetic	3	50–60
Assortment / **Nabisco** Pride	2.6	40–50
Creme, Swiss / **Nabisco**	2.5	40–50
Lemon / **Estee** Dietetic	3	40–50
Scotties / **Sunshine**	1.8	40–50

	FAT GRAMS	PERCENT OF CALORIES FROM FAT
Sesame cookies / **Stella D'Oro** Regina	2.2	40–50
Sesame cookies / **Stella D'Oro** Regina Dietetic	2.2	40–50
Shortbread / **Pepperidge Farm**	4	50–60
Shortbread, pecan / **Nabisco**	4.6	50–60
Social Tea Biscuit / **Nabisco**	.6	20–30
Social Tea Sandwich / **Nabisco**	2.2	30–40
Sorrento cookies / **Stella D'Oro** ..	2.7	40–50
Sprinkles / **Sunshine**	1.5	20–30
Sugar / **Pepperidge Farm**	2.3	30–40
Sugar / **Sunshine**	3.7	30–40
Sugar Rings / **Nabisco**	2.5	30–40
Sunflower Raisin / **Pepperidge Farm**	3	50–60
Swiss Fudge / **Stella D'Oro**	3.8	50–60
Tahiti / **Pepperidge Farm**	5.5	50–60
Taste of Vienna / **Stella D'Oro**	4.3	40–50
Toy cookies / **Sunshine**	.4	20–30
Vanilla Snaps / **Nabisco**	.8	50–60
Vanilla thins, dietetic / **Estee**	1	30–40
Vienna Finger sandwich / **Sunshine**	2.9	30–40
Wafers		
Assorted, dietetic / **Estee**	2	50–60
Brown edge / **Nabisco**	1.2	30–40
Chocolate, dietetic / **Estee**	1	30–40
Peanut butter-chocolate, dietetic / **Estee**	5.1	50–60
Spiced / **Nabisco**	1.1	20–30
Sugar / **Biscos**	.9	40–50
Sugar / **Sunshine**	1.8	30–40
Sugar, lemon / **Sunshine**	1.9	30–40
Vanilla, dietetic / **Estee**	1	30–40
Vanilla / **Sunshine**	.6	30–40
Yum Yums / **Sunshine**	3.2	30–40
Zanzibar / **Pepperidge Farm**	2.3	50–60
Zuzu Ginger Snaps / **Nabisco**	.4	20–30

COOKIE MIXES AND DOUGH

	FAT GRAMS	PERCENT OF CALORIES FROM FAT
Bar, date, mix, prepared: 1/32 of pkg / **Betty Crocker**	2	30–40
Bar, Vienna, mix, prepared: 1/24 pkg / **Betty Crocker**	5	50–60
Brownies		
Chocolate chip butterscotch, mix, prepared: 1/16 pkg / **Betty Crocker**	5	30–40
Fudge, mix, prepared: 1/24 pkg / **Betty Crocker** Family Size	4	20–30
Fudge, mix, prepared: 1/16 pkg / **Betty Crocker** Regular Size	4	20–30
Fudge, mix, prepared: 1/24 pkg / **Betty Crocker** Supreme	4	30–40
Fudge, mix, prepared: 1 brownie / **Duncan Hines** Double Fudge	5	30–40
Fudge, mix, prepared: 1½-in square / **Pillsbury**	2.5	30–40
Fudge, mix, prepared: 1½-in square / **Pillsbury** Family Size	3	30–40
Fudge, refrigerator, to bake: 1/16 pkg / **Pillsbury**	4	30–40
German chocolate, mix, prepared: 1/16 pkg / **Betty Crocker**	5	30–40
Walnut, mix, prepared: 1/16 pkg / **Betty Crocker**	6	30–40
Walnut, mix, prepared: 1/24 pkg / **Betty Crocker** Family Size	6	30–40
Walnut, mix prepared: 1½-in sq / **Pillsbury**	3.5	40–50
Walnut, mix, prepared: 1½-in sq / **Pillsbury** Family Size	3.5	40–50
Butterscotch nut, refrigerator, to bake: 1/36 pkg / **Pillsbury**	3	50–60

	FAT GRAMS	PERCENT OF CALORIES FROM FAT
Chocolate chip, mix, prepared: 1/36 pkg / **Betty Crocker** Big Batch	4	40–50
Chocolate chip, refrigerator, to bake: 1/36 pkg / **Pillsbury**	2.7	40–50
Fudge, refrigerator, to bake: 1/30 pkg / **Pillsbury**	3	30–40
Fudge chip, mix, prepared: 1 cookie (.4 oz) / **Quaker**	3.5	40–50
Ginger, refrigerator, to bake: 1/36 pkg / **Pillsbury Spicy**	1	10–20
Macaroon, coconut, mix, prepared: 1/24 pkg / **Betty Crocker**	4	40–50
Oatmeal, mix, prepared: 1/36 pkg / **Betty Crocker** Big Batch	3.5	40–50
Oatmeal, mix, prepared: 1 cookie (½ oz) / **Quaker**	3	40–50
Oatmeal chocolate chip, refrigerator, to bake: 1/36 pkg / **Pillsbury**	2.7	40–50
Oatmeal raisin, refrigerator, to bake: 1/36 pkg / **Pillsbury**	2.7	40–50
Peanut butter, mix, prepared: 1/36 pkg / **Betty Crocker** Big Batch	4	50–60
Peanut butter, mix, prepared: 1 cookie (.4 oz) **Quaker**	4.5	50–60
Peanut butter, refrigerator, to bake: 1/36 pkg / **Pillsbury**	3	50–60
Sugar, refrigerator, to bake: 1 cookie (1/36 pkg) / **Pillsbury**	3	40–50
Sugar, mix, prepared: 1/36 pkg / **Betty Crocker** Big Batch	3	40–50
Sugar, mix, prepared: 1 cookie (½ oz) / **Quaker**	4.5	40–50

Corn Starch

Corn starch has only trace amounts of fat.

Crackers

1 cracker unless noted	FAT GRAMS	PERCENT OF CALORIES FROM FAT
Cheez-Its: 1 piece / **Sunshine**	.3	40–50
Cheese filled: 1½ oz / **Frito-Lay**	9.5	40–50
Fling Curls / **Nabisco**	.7	60–70
Gold Fish		
Cheddar cheese: 1 oz / **Pepperidge Farm**	7	40–50
Lightly salted: 1 oz / **Pepperidge Farm**	6	40–50
Parmesan cheese: 1 oz / **Pepperidge Farm**	6	40–50
Pizza: 1 oz / **Pepperidge Farm**	7	40–50
Pretzel: 1 oz / **Pepperidge Farm**	3	20–30
Sesame-garlic: 1 oz / **Pepperidge Farm**	7	40–50
Taco: 1 oz / **Pepperidge Farm**	6	40–50
Thins, cheddar cheese: 4 thins / **Pepperidge Farm**	3	30–40
Thins, lightly salted: 4 thins / **Pepperidge Farm**	3	30–40
Thins, rye: 4 thins / **Pepperidge Farm**	3	30–40
Thins, wheat: 4 thins / **Pepperidge Farm**	4	50–60

	FAT GRAMS	PERCENT OF CALORIES FROM FAT
Hi Ho / **Sunshine**	1	50–60
Kavli Flatbread: 1 wafer	0	0–10
Matzos: 1 sheet or 1 cracker		
American / **Manischewitz**	1.9	10–20
Thins / **Manischewitz**	.4	0–10
Egg Matzo / **Manischewitz** Passover	.7	0–10
Egg 'n' Onion / **Manischewitz**	1	0–10
Onion Tams / **Manischewitz**	.6	40–50
Regular Matzo / **Manischewitz** Passover	.4	0–10
Tam Tams / **Manischewitz**	.7	40–50
Thin Tea / **Manischewitz**	.3	0–10
Whole Wheat / **Manischewitz**	.6	0–10
Mixed Suites, green onion: 1 oz / **Pepperidge Farm**	6	30–40
Mixed Suites, pretzel-cheese: 1 oz / **Pepperidge Farm**	3	20–30
Mixed Suites, sesame-cheese: 1 oz / **Pepperidge Farm**	7	40–50
Oyster / **Sunshine**	.1	30–40
Peanut butter: 1½ oz / **Frito-Lay**	10.6	40–60
Ritz / **Nabisco**	.8	40–50
Ritz Cheese / **Nabisco**	.1	0–10
Saltines and soda crackers		
Krispy / **Sunshine**	.2	10–20
Premium / **Nabisco**	.3	20–30
Premium, unsalted tops / **Nabisco**	.3	20–30
Royal Lunch / **Nabisco**	.3	0–10
Soda / **Sunshine**	.5	20–30
Uneeda, unsalted tops / **Nabisco**	.6	20–30
Shapies, cheese-flavored / **Nabisco**	.6	50–60
Shapies, cheese-flavored shells / **Nabisco**	.6	50–60
Sip 'N Chips, cheese-flavored / **Nabisco**	.5	50–60
Sociables / **Nabisco**	.4	50–60

	FAT GRAMS	PERCENT OF CALORIES FROM FAT
Triangle Thins / **Nabisco**	.3	30–40
Triscuit / **Nabisco**	.8	30–40
Twigs / **Nabisco**	.7	40–50
Waverly Wafers / **Nabisco**	.8	40–50
Wheat Thins / **Nabisco**	.4	40–50
Zwieback / **Nabisco**	.7	20–30

Cream

	FAT GRAMS	PERCENT OF CALORIES FROM FAT
1 tablespoon		
Medium cream (25% fat)	3.7	90–100
Light cream	2.9	80–90
Half-and-half	1.7	70–80
Sour cream	2.5	80–90
Whipped cream topping	.7	70–80
Heavy whipping cream (unwhipped)	5.5	90–100
Light whipping cream (unwhipped)	4.6	90–100

NON-DAIRY CREAMERS

Dry		
Carnation Coffee-Mate / 1 packet	1.1	50–60
Coffee Tone / 1 tsp	1	70–80
Cremora / 1 tsp	1	70–80

Liquid		
Coffee Rich: ½ oz	1	40–50
Coffee Tone Freezer Pack / 1 tbsp	2	80–90
Lucerne Cereal Blend / ½ cup	12	70–80

Dessert Mixes

	FAT GRAMS	PERCENT OF CALORIES FROM FAT
Apple cinnamon, mix, prepared: ⅔ cup / **Pillsbury** Appleasy	3	10–20
Apple caramel, prepared: ½ cup / **Pillsbury** Appleasy	2	10–20
Apple raisin, prepared: ⅔ cup / **Pillsbury** Appleasy	3	10–20

Diet Bars

	FAT GRAMS	PERCENT OF CALORIES FROM FAT
All flavors: 1 bar / **Pillsbury** Figurines	8	50–60
All flavors: 1 stick / **Pillsbury** Food Sticks	1.5	30–40
Cinnamon: 1 bar / **Carnation** Slender Bars	7	40–50
Chocolate: 1 bar / **Carnation** Slender Bars	8	50–60
Vanilla: 1 bar / **Carnation** Slender Bars	7	40–50

Dinners

FROZEN DINNERS

	FAT GRAMS	PERCENT OF CALORIES FROM FAT
1 dinner		
Beans and beef patties: 11 oz / **Swanson "TV"**	17	10–20
Beans and franks: 10¾ oz / **Banquet**	30.2	40–50
Beans and franks: 10¾ oz / **Morton**	17	20–30
Beans and franks: 11¼ oz / **Swanson "TV"**	20	30–40
Beef		
Banquet / 11 oz	11.9	30–40
La Choy	7	10–20
Morton / 10 oz	11	30–40
Swanson 3 Course / 15 oz	17	30–40
Swanson "TV" / 11½ oz	12	20–30
Beef, chopped: 11 oz / **Banquet**	26.5	50–60
Beef, chopped: 11 oz / **Morton**	22	50–60
Beef, sirloin chopped: 10 oz / **Swanson "TV"**	25	40–50
Beef, sirloin chopped: 16 oz / **Weight Watchers**	37	50–60
Beef, sliced: 14 oz / **Morton** Country Table	20	30–40
Beef, sliced: 17 oz / **Swanson** Hungry-Man	18	30–40
Beef steak, chopped: 18 oz / **Swanson** Hungry-Man	41	50–60
Beef steak, chopped: 10 oz / **Weight Watchers**	24	50–60
Beef tenderloin: 9½ oz / **Morton** Steak House Dinner	65	60–70

	FAT GRAMS	PERCENT OF CALORIES FROM FAT
Chicken / **La Choy**	8	20–30
Chicken, boneless: 10 oz / **Morton**	7	20–30
Chicken, boneless: 19 oz / **Swanson** Hungry-Man	29	30–40
Chicken breast: 15 oz / **Weight Watchers**	7	10–20
Chicken croquette: 10¼ oz / **Morton**	18	30–40
Chicken, fried		
Banquet / 11 oz	25	40–50
Banquet Man Pleaser / 17 oz	51.6	40–50
Morton / 11 oz	14	20–30
Morton Country Table / 15 oz	18	20–30
Swanson Hungry-Man / 15¾ oz	46	40–50
Swanson Hungry-Man Barbecue-flavored / 16½ oz	35	40–50
Swanson 3 Course / 15 oz	31	40–50
Swanson "TV" / 11½ oz	29	40–50
Barbecue-flavored: 11¼ oz / **Swanson** "TV"	26	40–50
Crispy fried: 10¾ oz / **Swanson** "TV"	34	40–50
Chicken and dumplings: 12 oz / **Banquet**	8.2	20–30
Chicken w dumplings: 11 oz / **Morton**	10	30–40
Chicken and noodles: 12 oz / **Banquet**	10.5	20–30
Chicken w noodles: 10¼ oz / **Morton**	7	20–30
Chicken oriental style: 15 oz / **Weight Watchers**	6	10–20
Chop suey, beef: 12 oz / **Banquet**	8.2	20–30
Chow mein, chicken: 12 oz / **Banquet**	12.2	30–40
Enchilada, beef: 12 oz / **Banquet**	17.3	30–40
Enchilada, beef: 15 oz / **Swanson** "TV"	23	30–40
Enchilada, cheese: 12 oz / **Banquet**	16.7	30–40
Fish: 8¾ oz / **Banquet**	14.6	30–40

	FAT GRAMS	PERCENT OF CALORIES FROM FAT
Fish: 9 oz / **Morton**	9	30–40
Fish 'n' Chips: 15¾ oz / **Swanson** Hungry-Man	35	40–50
Fish 'n' Chips: 10¼ oz / **Swanson** "TV"	20	40–50
Flounder: 16 oz / **Weight Watchers**	3	10–20
German Style: 11¾ oz / **Swanson** "TV"	17	30–40
Haddock: 8¾ oz / **Banquet**	16.9	30–40
Haddock: 16 oz / **Weight Watchers**	2	0–10
Ham: 10 oz / **Banquet**	12.2	20–30
Ham: 10 oz / **Morton**	17	30–40
Ham: 10¼ oz / **Swanson** "TV"	13	30–40
Hash, corned beef: 10 oz / **Banquet**	13.3	30–40
Italian Style: 11 oz / **Banquet**	20.9	40–50
Italian Style: 13 oz / **Swanson** "TV"	17	30–40
Lasagna w meat: 17¾ oz / **Swanson** Hungry-Man	32	30–40
Macaroni and beef: 12 oz / **Banquet**	13.6	30–40
Macaroni and beef: 10 oz / **Morton**	5	10–20
Macaroni and beef: 12 oz / **Swanson** "TV"	15	30–40
Macaroni and cheese: 12 oz / **Banquet**	10.2	20–30
Macaroni and cheese: 11 oz / **Morton**	9	20–30
Macaroni and cheese: 12½ oz / **Swanson** "TV"	14	30–40
Meat loaf: 11 oz / **Banquet**	23.7	50–60
Meat loaf: 11 oz / **Morton**	15	30–40
Meat loaf: 15 oz / **Morton** Country Table	16	30–40
Meat loaf: 10¾ oz / **Swanson** "TV"	29	40–50
Meatballs: 11¾ oz / **Swanson** "TV"	24	50–60
Mexican style: 16 oz / **Banquet**	25.4	30–40
Mexican style combination: 12 oz / **Banquet**	21.4	30–40

	FAT GRAMS	PERCENT OF CALORIES FROM FAT
Mexican style combination: 16 oz / **Swanson "TV"**	25	30–40
Noodles and chicken: 10¼ oz / **Swanson "TV"**	15	30–40
Pepper oriental / **La Choy**	7	10–20
Perch, ocean: 8¾ oz / **Banquet**	17.6	30–40
Perch, ocean: 16 oz / **Weight Watchers**	11	30–40
Polynesian style: 13 oz / **Swanson "TV"**	17	30–40
Pork, loin of: 11¼ oz / **Swanson "TV"**	22	40–50
Rib eye: 9 oz / **Morton** Steak House Dinner	58	60–70
Salisbury steak		
Banquet / 11 oz	24.6	50–60
Morton / 11 oz	13	40–50
Morton Country Table / 15 oz	15	30–40
Swanson Hungry-Man / 17 oz	52	50–60
Swanson 3 Course / 16 oz	24	40–50
Swanson "TV" / 11½ oz	29	50–60
Shrimp / **La Choy**	6	10–20
Sirloin, chopped: 9½ oz / **Morton** Steak House Dinner	47	50–60
Sirloin strip: 9½ oz / **Morton** Steak House Dinner	65	60–70
Sole: 16 oz / **Weight Watchers**	3	10–20
Spaghetti and meatballs: 11½ oz / **Banquet**	15.3	30–40
Spaghetti and meatballs: 11 oz / **Morton**	8	20–30
Spaghetti and meatballs: 18½ oz / **Swanson** Hungry-Man	26	30–40
Spaghetti and meatballs: 12½ oz / **Swanson "TV"**	14	30–40
Swiss steak: 10 oz / **Swanson "TV"**	13	30–40

	FAT GRAMS	PERCENT OF CALORIES FROM FAT
Turbot: 16 oz / **Weight Watchers**	22	40–50
Turkey		
Banquet / 11 oz	9.7	20–30
Banquet Man-Pleaser / 19 oz	18.9	20–30
Morton / 11 oz	14	30–40
Morton Country Table / 15 oz	17	20–30
Swanson Hungry-Man / 19 oz	25	30–40
Swanson 3 Course / 16 oz	21	30–40
Swanson "TV" / 11½ oz	11	20–30
Breast: 16 oz / **Weight Watchers**	12	20–30
Veal Parmagian: 11 oz / **Banquet**	19	40–50
Veal Parmigiana: 10¼ oz / **Morton**	9	20–30
Veal Parmigiana: 20½ oz / **Swanson** Hungry-Man	53	50–60
Veal Parmigiana: 12¼ oz / **Swanson** "TV"	27	40–50
Western: 11 oz / **Banquet**	24	50–60
Western Round-Up: 11¾ oz / **Morton**	23	50–60
Western Style: 17¾ oz / **Swanson** Hungry-Man	42	40–50
Western Style: 11¾ oz / **Swanson** "TV"	22	40–50

DINNER MIXES

	FAT GRAMS	PERCENT OF CALORIES FROM FAT
Ann Page Beef Noodle Dinner: 1/5 prepared dinner	16	40–50
Ann Page Cheeseburger Macaroni Dinner: 1/5 prepared dinner	18	40–50
Ann Page Chili Tomato Dinner: 1.6 oz before preparation	1	0–10
Ann Page Hash Dinner: 1/5 prepared dinner	14	40–50
Ann Page Italian Style Dinner: 2 oz before preparation	3	10–20

	FAT GRAMS	PERCENT OF CALORIES FROM FAT
Ann Page Potato Stroganoff Dinner: 1/5 prepared dinner	14	30–40
Hamburger Helper, Beef Noodle: 1/5 prepared dinner / **Betty Crocker**	15	40–50
Hamburger Helper, Beef Romanoff: 1/5 prepared dinner / **Betty Crocker**	16	40–50
Hamburger Helper, Cheeseburger Macaroni: 1/5 prepared dinner / **Betty Crocker**	18	40–50
Hamburger Helper, Chili Tomato: 1/5 prepared dinner / **Betty Crocker**	15	40–50
Hamburger Helper, Hamburger Hash: 1/5 prepared dinner / **Betty Crocker**	15	40–50
Hamburger Helper, Hamburger Pizza Dish: 1/5 prepared dinner / **Betty Crocker**	14	40–50
Hamburger Helper, Hamburger Stew: 1/5 prepared dinner / **Betty Crocker**	14	40–50
Hamburger Helper, Lasagna: 1/5 prepared dinner / **Betty Crocker**	14	30–40
Hamburger Helper, Potato Stroganoff: 1/5 prepared dinner / **Betty Crocker**	15	40–50
Hamburger Helper, Rice Oriental: 1/5 prepared dinner (8 oz pkg) / **Betty Crocker**	14	30–40
Hamburger Helper, Rice Oriental: 1/5 prepared dinner (6½ oz pkg) / **Betty Crocker**	13	20–30

	FAT GRAMS	PERCENT OF CALORIES FROM FAT
Hamburger Helper, Spaghetti: 1/5 prepared dinner / **Betty Crocker**	14	30–40
Tuna Helper, Dumplings and noodles: 1/5 prepared dinner / **Betty Crocker**	6	20–30
Tuna Helper, Noodles: 1/5 prepared dinner / **Betty Crocker**	11	30–40
Tuna Helper, Noodles w cheese sauce: 1/5 prepared dinner / **Betty Crocker**	7	20–30

Eggs

	FAT GRAMS	PERCENT OF CALORIES FROM FAT
Fresh		
Chicken egg		
Raw, hard-cooked or poached		
Extra large	6.6	60–70
Large	5.8	60–70
Medium	5.1	60–70
Raw, white only		
Extra large	trace	0–10
Large	trace	0–10
Medium	trace	0–10
One cup	.1	0–10
Raw, yolk only		
Extra large	5.8	70–80
Large	5.2	70–80
Medium	4.6	70–80
Fried		
Extra large	8.9	70–80
Large	7.9	70–80
Medium	6.9	70–80
Hard boiled, chopped: 1 cup	15.6	60–70
Duck, raw: 1 egg	10.2	60–70
Goose, raw: 1 egg	19.1	60–70
Turkey, raw: 1 egg	10.4	60–70

EGG MIXES AND SEASONINGS

	FAT GRAMS	PERCENT OF CALORIES FROM FAT
Egg, imitation, frozen: ¼ cup / Morningstar Farms Scramblers	3.1	40–50
Egg, imitation, mix: ½ pkg / Eggstra	2	30–40
Egg, imitation, refrigerated: ¼ cup / No-Fat Egg Beaters	0	0
Omelet, bacon, prepared: 1 pkg / Durkee	46	60–70
dry mix: 1 pkg	2	10–20
Omelet, cheese, prepared: 1 pkg / Durkee	51	70–80
dry mix: 1 pkg	7	50–60
Omelet, prepared: 1 pkg / Durkee Puffy	44	60–70
dry mix: 1 pkg	5	40–50
Omelet, Western: 1 pkg / Durkee (add water only to dehydrated eggs)	5	20–30
Omelet, Western, prepared: 1 pkg / Durkee (add fresh eggs)	44	60–70
dry mix: 1 pkg	.7	0–10
Scrambled: 1 pkg / Durkee (add water only)	10	70–80
Scrambled w bacon: 1 pkg / Durkee (add water only)	13	60–70

Fish and Seafood

The information was not available to accurately calculate the percentage of calories from fat for fresh fish and seafood. However, fish and seafood, with the exception of anchovies and eel, are generally very low in fat, deriving less than 20 percent of their calories from fat.

FRESH

	FAT GRAMS	PERCENT OF CALORIES FROM FAT
raw: 1 oz		
Anchovy	1.8	
Argentine, Atlantic, fillet	.1	
Bass, striped, fillet	.6	
Burbot, fillet	.3	
Carp, fillet	1.2	
Catfish, channel, fillet	1	
Cisco, fillet	.7	
Cod, fillet	.2	
Dogfish, fillet	2.8	
Eel, American, fillet	5.2	
Eel, European, fillet	7	
Flounder, yellowtail, fillet	.3	
Haddock, fillet	.2	
Hake, Pacific, fillet	.4	
Hake, silver, fillet	1	
Halibut, Atlantic, fillet	.3	
Halibut, Pacific, fillet	.6	

	FAT GRAMS	PERCENT OF CALORIES FROM FAT
Herring, fillet	1.8	
Mackerel, Atlantic, fillet	2.8	
Mullet, striped	1.7	
Ocean perch, fillet	.7	
Oilfish, fillet	4.2	
Pike, northern, fillet	.2	
Pilchard, fillet	1.9	
Pollock, fillet	.3	
Pomfret, silver, fillet	1.3	
Rabbitfish, fillet	.4	
Rockfish, fillet	.4	
Sablefish, fillet	3.7	
Salmon, Atlantic, fillet	1.6	
Salmon, chinnok, fillet	3.7	
Salmon, chum, fillet	1.1	
Salmon, Coho, fillet (Pacific)	2.1	
Salmon, coho, steak (Lake Michigan)	1.4	
Salmon, pink, fillet	1.5	
Salmon, sockeye, fillet	2.5	
Sand lance, whole	2	
Scad, fillet	.7	
Sea bass, Japanese, fillet	.8	
Shark, salmon	.5	
Smelt, rainbow	.5	
Snapper, red, fillet	.3	
Sole, fillet	.2	
Sprat, whole	3.8	
Sprat, fillet	1.4	
Sturgeon, common, fillet	.9	
Sturgeon, Russian, fillet	3	
Trout, brook, whole eviscerated	2.2	
Trout, rainbow, European, fillet	1.3	
Trout, rainbow, U.S. fillet	1.3	
Tuna, albacore, white meat	2.3	
Tuna, bluefin, fillet	1.3	
Turbot	2.4	

	FAT GRAMS	PERCENT OF CALORIES FROM FAT
Whitefish, lake, fillet	1.5	
Wolffish, fillet	.8	
Wrasse, fillet	.6	
Yellowtail, fillet	1.5	

SHELLFISH

	FAT GRAMS	PERCENT OF CALORIES FROM FAT
Abalone	.3	
Clam	.4	
Crab, Alaska King, cooked, legs and claws	.5	
Crab, blue, cooked	.5	
Crab, Dungeness, meat	.3	
Lobster, Caribbean	.3	
Lobster, rock, tail meat	.3	
Mussel	.5	
Octopus	.2	
Oyster, Eastern and Pacific	.6	
Periwinkle	1	
Scallop	.2	
Shrimp	.3	
Snail, pond	.8	
Squid	.6	

CANNED AND FROZEN

	FAT GRAMS	PERCENT OF CALORIES FROM FAT
Clams		
Chopped or minced, canned: ½ cup / **Snow's**	0	0–10
Fried, frozen: 5 oz / **Howard Johnson's**	13.9	30–40
Fried, frozen: 2½ oz / **Mrs. Paul's**	16	50–60
Cakes, frozen: 1 cake / **Mrs. Paul's** Thins	7	40–50
Deviled, frozen: 1 cake / **Mrs. Paul's**	10	50–60

	FAT GRAMS	PERCENT OF CALORIES FROM FAT
Sticks, frozen: 1 stick / **Mrs. Paul's**	1.4	20–30
Crab cakes, frozen: 1 cake / **Mrs. Paul's** Thins	7.5	40–50
Crabs, deviled, frozen: 1 cake / **Mrs. Paul's**	7	30–40
Crabs, deviled, frozen: 3½ oz / **Mrs. Paul's** Miniatures	9	20–30
Fish, frozen		
Cakes: 1 cake / **Mrs. Paul's**	4	30–40
Cakes: 1 cake / **Mrs. Paul's** Beach Haven	3.5	20–30
Cakes: 1 cake / **Mrs. Paul's** Thins	9	50–60
In light batter: 3 oz / **Mrs. Paul's** Miniatures	5	30–40
Fillets, buttered: 1 fillet (2½ oz) / **Mrs. Paul's**	13	70–80
Fillets, fried: 1 fillet (2 oz) / **Mrs. Paul's**	4.5	30–40
Fillets, in light batter: 1 fillet / **Mrs. Paul's**	6.5	40–50
Fillets, in light batter, fried: 1 fillet / **Mrs. Paul's** Supreme	10	40–50
Sticks: 1 stick / **Mrs. Paul's**	1.3	30–40
Sticks, in light batter, fried: 1 stick / **Mrs. Paul's**	2.5	30–40
Flounder, fried, frozen: 1 fillet (2 oz) / **Mrs. Paul's**	5	40–50
Flounder w lemon butter, frozen: 4½ oz / **Mrs. Paul's**	8	40–50
Gefilte fish, in jars: 1 piece		
Homestyle, (4-piece, 12 oz jar) / **Manischewitz**	3.3	50–60
Homestyle, (8-piece, 24 oz jar) / **Manischewitz**	3.3	50–60

	FAT GRAMS	PERCENT OF CALORIES FROM FAT
Homestyle, (24-piece, 4 lb jar) / **Manischewitz**	3	50–60
Regular, (4-piece, 12 oz jar) / **Manischewitz**	3.3	50–60
Regular, (8- piece, 24 oz jar) / **Manischewitz**	3.3	50–60
Regular, (24-piece, 4 lb jar) / **Manischewitz**	2.9	50–60
Sweet, (4-piece, 12 oz jar) / **Manischewitz**	3.7	50–60
Sweet, (8-piece, 24 oz jar) / **Manischewitz**	3.7	50–60
Sweet, (24-piece, 4 lb jar) / **Manischewitz**	3.3	50–60
Fishlets, (55-piece, 24 oz jar) / **Manischewitz**	.5	50–60
Whitefish and pike, (4-piece, 12 oz jar) / **Manischewitz**	3.1	50–60
Whitefish and pike, (8-piece, 24 oz jar) / **Manischewitz**	3.1	50–60
Whitefish and pike, (24-piece, 4 lb jar) / **Manischewitz**	2.7	50–60
Whitefish and pike, sweet, (4-piece, 12 oz jar) / **Manischewitz**	3.4	50–60
Whitefish and pike, sweet, (8-piece, 24 oz jar) / **Manischewitz**	3.4	50–60
Whitefish and pike, sweet, (24-piece, 4 lb jar) / **Manischewitz**	3.1	50–60
Haddock, fried, frozen: 1 fillet (2 oz) / **Mrs. Paul's**	4.5	30–40
Oysters, without shell, canned: ½ can / **Bumblebee**	2.5	20–30
Perch, fried, frozen: 1 fillet (2 oz) / **Mrs. Paul's**	7	50–60
Salmon, canned Pink: 7¾ oz / **Del Monte**	13	30–40

	FAT GRAMS	PERCENT OF CALORIES FROM FAT
Red sockeye: ½ cup / **Bumblebee**	7.8	40–50
Red sockeye: 7¾ oz / **Del Monte**	17	40–50
Sardines, in mustard sauce: 1 oz / **Underwood**	3.8	60–70
Sardines, in soya bean oil: 1 oz / **Underwood**	4.3	60–70
Sardines, in tomato sauce, canned: 1 oz / **Del Monte**	2.4	40–50
Sardines, in tomato sauce: 1 oz / **Underwood**	2.6	50–60
Scallops, fried, frozen: 3½ oz / **Mrs. Paul's**	8	30–40
Scallops, in light batter, fried, frozen: 3½ oz / **Mrs. Paul's**	8	30–40
Seafood, combination, fried, frozen: 9 oz / **Mrs. Paul's** Platter	22	30–40
Seafood croquettes, frozen: 1 cake / **Mrs. Paul's**	6	30–40
Shrimp		
Baby, solids and liquids: one 4½ oz can / **Bumblebee**	.9	0–10
In cocktail sauce: 4 oz jar / **Sau-Sea** Shrimp Cocktail	.6	0–10
Frozen, in bag, cooked: 2 oz / **Sau-Sea**	.3	0–10
Fried, frozen: 3 oz / **Mrs. Paul's**	11	50–60
Fried, frozen: 4 oz / **Sau-Sea** Shrimp Fries	10	30–40
Cakes, frozen: 1 cake / **Mrs. Paul's**	5	30–40
Cakes, frozen: 1 cake / **Mrs. Paul's** Thins	7	40–50
Sticks, frozen: 1 stick / **Mrs. Paul's**	2	30–40
Sole w lemon butter, frozen: 4½ oz / **Mrs. Paul's**	8	40–50
Tuna, canned		
In oil, drained: ½ cup / **Bumblebee**	6.9	30–40

	FAT GRAMS	PERCENT OF CALORIES FROM FAT
In water, undrained: ½ cup / **Bumblebee**	2.5	0–10
Light chunk, in oil: 6½ oz / **Del Monte**	29	50–60

FROZEN ENTREES

	FAT GRAMS	PERCENT OF CALORIES FROM FAT
Crepes, clam: 5½ oz / **Mrs. Paul's**	17	50–60
Crepes, crab: 5½ oz / **Mrs. Paul's**	12	40–50
Crepes, scallop: 5½ oz / **Mrs. Paul's**	9	30–40
Crepes, shrimp: 5½ oz / **Mrs. Paul's**	12	40–50
Croquette, shrimp w Newburg sauce: 12 oz / **Howard Johnson's**	38	70–80
Fish au gratin: 5 oz / **Mrs. Paul's**	12	40–50
Fish au gratin: 4 oz / **Mrs. Paul's** Party Pak	11	40–50
Fish 'n' Chips: 1 entree / **Swanson "TV"**	14	40–50
Fish 'n Chips, in light batter, fried: 7 oz / **Mrs. Paul's**	16	30–40
Fish Parmesan: 5 oz / **Mrs. Paul's**	11	40–50
Fish Parmesan: 4 oz / **Mrs. Paul's** Party Pak	8	40–50
Flounder w chopped broccoli, cauliflower, red peppers: 8½ oz / **Weight Watchers**	2	10–20
Haddock au Groton: 10 oz / **Howard Johnson's**	14.3	40–50
Haddock w stuffing and spinach: 8¾ oz / **Weight Watchers**	2	10–20
Perch, ocean w chopped broccoli: 8½ oz / **Weight Watchers**	5	20–30
Scallops w butter and cheese: 7 oz / **Mrs. Paul's**	12	40–50
Shrimp and Scallops Mariner: 10¼ oz pkg / **Stouffer's**	16	30–40

	FAT GRAMS	PERCENT OF CALORIES FROM FAT
Sole w peas, mushrooms, and lobster sauce: 9½ oz / **Weight Watchers**	3	10–20
Tuna, creamed w peas: 5 oz / **Green Giant** Boil-in-Bag Toast Toppers	8	50–60
Turbot w peas and carrots: 8 oz / **Weight Watchers**	15	40–50

Flavorings, Sweet

No fat

Flour, Meal and Grains

FLOUR

	FAT GRAMS	PERCENT OF CALORIES FROM FAT
1 cup unless noted		
Biscuit mix / **Bisquick**	16	30–40
Buckwheat, dark, sifted	2.5	0–10
Buckwheat, light, sifted	1.2	0–10

	FAT GRAMS	PERCENT OF CALORIES FROM FAT
Carob	2	0–10
Corn	3	0–10
Lima bean flour, sifted	1.8	0–10
Peanut flour, defatted	5.5	20–30
Rye		
Light	.9	0–10
Medium	1.5	0–10
Dark	3.3	0–10
Rye, medium / **Pillsbury**	3	0–10
Rye wheat / **Pillsbury** Bohemian	1	0–10
Soybean		
Full fat	14.2	40–50
Low fat	5.9	10–20
Defatted	.9	0–10
Tortilla, corn: ⅓ cup / **Quaker's**		
Masa Harina	1.5	0–10
Tortilla, wheat: ⅓ cup / **Quaker's**		
Masa Trigo	4	20–30
Wheat		
All purpose	1.4	0–10
Bread	1.5	0–10
Cake or pastry	.9	0–10
Gluten	2.7	0–10
Self-rising	1.3	0–10
Whole wheat	2.4	0–10
Whole wheat / **Pillsbury**	2	0–10
White		
Ballard	1	0–10
Pillsbury, all purpose	1	0–10
Cake, self rising / **Presto**	.9	0–10
Self-rising: ¼ cup / **Aunt Jemima**	.3	0–10
Self-rising / **Ballard**	1	0–10
Self-rising / **Pillsbury**	1	0–10
Unbleached / **Pillsbury**	1	0–10

MEAL

	FAT GRAMS	PERCENT OF CALORIES FROM FAT
Almond meal, partially defatted: 1 oz	5.2	40–50
Corn, white or yellow, whole ground unbolted, dry: 1 cup	4.8	0–10
Crackermeal: 1 cup / **Sunshine**	1.1	0–10

GRAINS

	FAT GRAMS	PERCENT OF CALORIES FROM FAT
Bulgur wheat, dry: 1 cup		
Made from club wheat	2.5	0–10
Made from hard winter wheat	2.6	0–10
Made from white wheat	1.9	0–10

Frostings

	FAT GRAMS	PERCENT OF CALORIES FROM FAT
Ready to Spread: 1 can unless noted		
Cake and cookie decorator, all colors:		
1 tbsp / **Pillsbury**	2	20–30
Butter pecan / **Betty Crocker**	84	30–40
Cherry / **Betty Crocker**	72	30–40
Chocolate / **Betty Crocker**	96	40–50
Chocolate fudge / **Pillsbury**	84	30–40
Chocolate nut / **Betty Crocker**	84	30–40
Dark Dutch fudge / **Betty Crocker**	84	30–40
Double Dutch / **Pillsbury**	84	30–40
Lemon / **Betty Crocker** Sunkist	72	30–40
Lemon / **Pillsbury**	72	30–40

	FAT GRAMS	PERCENT OF CALORIES FROM FAT
Milk chocolate / **Betty Crocker**	84	30–40
Milk chocolate / **Pillsbury**	84	30–40
Orange / **Betty Crocker**	72	30–40
Sour cream, chocolate /		
Betty Crocker	96	40–50
Sour cream, vanilla / **Pillsbury**	72	30–40
Sour cream, white / **Betty Crocker**	72	30–40
Strawberry / **Pillsbury**	72	30–40
Vanilla / **Betty Crocker**	72	30–40
Vanilla / **Pillsbury**	72	30–40

1 pkg: prepared

	FAT GRAMS	PERCENT OF CALORIES FROM FAT
Banana / **Betty Crocker** Chiquita	36	10–20
Butter Brickle / **Betty Crocker**	36	10–20
Butter pecan / **Betty Crocker**	36	10–20
Caramel / **Pillsbury** Rich 'n Easy	72	30–40
Cherry / **Betty Crocker**	36	10–20
Chocolate / **Betty Crocker** Lite	36	20–30
Chocolate fudge / **Betty Crocker**	36	10–20
Chocolate fudge / **Pillsbury**		
Rich 'n Easy	60	20–30
Coconut almond / **Pillsbury**	120	50–60
Coconut pecan / **Betty Crocker**	48	30–40
Coconut pecan / **Pillsbury**	96	40–50
Dark chocolate fudge / **Betty Crocker**	36	10–20
Double Dutch / **Pillsbury**		
Rich 'n Easy	60	20–30
Lemon / **Betty Crocker** Sunkist	36	10–20
Lemon / **Pillsbury** Rich 'n Easy	60	20–30
Milk chocolate / **Betty Crocker**	36	10–20
Milk chocolate / **Pillsbury**		
Rich 'n Easy	72	30–40
Sour cream, chocolate /		
Betty Crocker	36	10–20
Sour cream, white / **Betty Crocker**	36	10–20
Strawberry / **Pillsbury** Rich 'n Easy	72	30–40

	FAT GRAMS	PERCENT OF CALORIES FROM FAT
Vanilla / **Betty Crocker** Lite	36	20–30
Vanilla / **Pillsbury** Rich 'n Easy	72	30–40
White, creamy / **Betty Crocker**	36	10–20
White, fluffy / **Betty Crocker** Lite	0	0
White, fluffy / **Pillsbury**	0	0

Fruit

FRESH

	FAT GRAMS	PERCENT OF CALORIES FROM FAT
Apples w skin: 1 large	1.3	0–10
Apple w skin: 1 small	.6	0–10
Apple, peeled: 1 large	.6	0–10
Apricots, raw, whole: 3 apricots	.2	0–10
Avocados, California: ½ average size	18.4	80–90
Avocados, California, cubed: 1 cup	25.5	80–90
Avocados, California, puree: 1 cup	39.1	80–90
Avocados, Florida: ½ average size	16.8	70–80
Avocados, Florida, cubed: 1 cup	16.5	70–80
Avocados, Florida, puree: 1 cup	25.3	70–80
Banana: 1 large	.3	0–10
Blackberries: 1 cup	1.3	10–20
Blueberries: 1 cup	.7	0–10
Cherries: 1 cup	.3	0–10
Cranberries, raw, whole: 1 cup	.7	10–20
Fig, raw, whole: 1 fig	.2	0–10
Grapefruit: half, 3½-in diam	.1	0–10

	FAT GRAMS	PERCENT OF CALORIES FROM FAT
Grapes: 10 grapes	.3	0–10
Lemons: 1 large	.3	0–10
Lime: 1 lime	.1	0–10
Mangos, raw, whole: 1 fruit	.9	0–10
Muskmelons, canteloupe: half, 5-in diam	.3	0–10
Nectarine: 1 nectarine	trace	0–10
Orange: 1 large	.2	0–10
Papaya: 1 papaya	.3	0–10
Peach: 1 large	.2	0–10
Pear: 1 pear	.7	0–10
Pineapple, raw, diced: 1 cup	.3	0–10
Plums, raw, whole: 10 plums	trace	0–10
Raspberries, raw, black: 1 cup	1.9	10–20
Raspberries, raw, red: 1 cup	.6	0–10
Rhubarb, diced, raw: 1 cup	.1	0–10
Strawberries, raw, whole berries: 1 cup	.7	10–20
Tangerines: 1 large	.2	0–10
Watermelon, raw, diced pieces: 1 cup	.3	0–10

Fruits and Fruit Juices and Drinks

Canned, frozen, dried: Negligible amounts of fat anywhere from zero to 1 gram per serving

		PERCENT OF
	FAT	CALORIES
	GRAMS	FROM FAT

Gelatin

No fat

Gravies

	FAT GRAMS	PERCENT OF CALORIES FROM FAT
Au jus		
Mix, prepared: 1 env / **Ann Page**	0	0–10
Mix, prepared: ¼ cup / **Durkee**	.7	0–10
Mix w roasting bag: 1 pkg / **Durkee**		
Roastin' Bag	1	10–20
Mix, prepared: ¼ cup / **French's**	0	0–10
Mix, prepared: ¼ cup / **French's**		
Pan Rich	2	60–70
Beef, canned: 1/5 can / **Ann Page**	1	30–40
Beef, canned: 2 oz / **Franco-American**	1	30–40
Beef, canned: ½ cup /		
Howard Johnson's	2.5	40–50
Brown		
Mix, prepared: 1 env / **Ann Page**	4	40–50
Mix, prepared: ¼ cup / **Durkee**	.1	0–10
Mix, prepared: ¼ cup / **French's**	1	40–50

	FAT GRAMS	PERCENT OF CALORIES FROM FAT
Mix, prepared: ¼ cup / **French's** Pan Rich	5	70–80
Mix, prepared: ¼ cup / **Pillsbury**	0	0–10
Mix, prepared: 1 fl oz / **Spatini** Family Style	0	0–10
Mix, prepared: ¼ cup / **Weight Watchers**	0	0–10
w mushroom broth, canned: 1 oz / **Dawn Fresh**	.5	40–50
w mushroom, mix, prepared: ¼ cup / **Durkee**	.1	0–10
w mushrooms, mix, prepared: ¼ cup / **Weight Watchers**	0	0–10
w onions, canned: 2 oz / **Franco-American**	1	30–40
w onions, mix, prepared: ¼ cup / **Durkee**	.1	0–10
w onions, mix, prepared: ¼ cup / **Weight Watchers**	0	0–10
Chicken		
Canned: 2 oz / **Franco American**	4	70–80
Mix, prepared: 1 env / **Ann Page**	4	30–40
Mix, prepared: ¼ cup / **Durkee**	.6	20–30
Mix, prepared: ¼ cup / **Durkee** Creamy	2.2	50–60
Mix, prepared: ¼ cup / **French's**	1	30–40
Mix, prepared: ¼ cup / **French's** Pan Rich	5	70–80
Mix, prepared: ¼ cup / **Pillsbury**	1	30–40
Mix, prepared: ¼ cup / **Weight Watchers**	0	0–10
Mix w roasting bag: 1 pkg / **Durkee** Roastin' Bag	1	0–10
Mix w roasting bag: 1 pkg /**Durkee** Roastin' Bag Italian style	1	0–10

	FAT GRAMS	PERCENT OF CALORIES FROM FAT
Creamy, mix, w roasting bag:		
1 pkg / **Durkee** Roastin' Bag	12	40–50
Chicken giblet, canned: 2 oz /		
Franco-American	2	50–60
Homestyle, mix, prepared: ¼ cup /		
Durkee	.5	20–30
Homestyle, mix, prepared: ¼ cup /		
French's	1	30–40
Homestyle, mix, prepared: ¼ cup /		
Pillsbury	0	0–10
Meatloaf, mix w roasting bag: 1 pkg /		
Durkee Roastin' Bag	1	0–10
Mushroom		
Canned: 2 oz / **Franco-American**	2	50–60
Mix, prepared: 1 env / **Ann Page**	4	40–50
Mix, prepared: ¼ cup / **French's**	1	40–50
Onion, mix, prepared:		
1 env / **Ann Page**	4	30–40
Onion, mix, prepared: ¼ cup /		
Durkee	.1	0–10
Onion, mix, prepared: ¼ cup /		
French's	1	30–40
Onion, mix, prepared: ¼ cup /		
French's Pan Rich	4	70–80
Onion pot roast, mix w roasting bag:		
1 pkg / **Durkee** Roastin' Bag	.1	0–10
Pork, mix, prepared: ¼ cup / **Durkee**	.1	0–10
Pork, mix, prepared: ¼ cup / **French's**	1	40–50
Pork, mix w roasting bag: 1 pkg /		
Durkee Roastin' Bag	1	0–10
Pot roast stew, mix w roasting bag:		
1 pkg / **Durkee** Roastin' Bag	1	0–10
Sparerib sauce, mix w roasting bag:		
1 pkg / **Durkee** Roastin' Bag	2	0–10
Swiss steak, mix, prepared: ¼ cup /		
Durkee	.1	0–10

	FAT GRAMS	PERCENT OF CALORIES FROM FAT
Swiss steak, mix w roasting bag: 1 pkg / **Durkee** Roastin' Bag	.9	0–10
Turkey giblet, canned: ½ cup / **Howard Johnson's**	3.4	50–60
Turkey, mix, prepared: ¼ cup / **Durkee**	.5	10–20
Turkey, mix, prepared: ¼ cup / **French's**	1	30–40

Health Foods

	FAT GRAMS	PERCENT OF CALORIES FROM FAT
Granola Bars		
w cinnamon: 1 bar / **Nature Valley**	4	30–40
w coconut: 1 bar / **Nature Valley**	6	40–50
w oats and honey: 1 bar /		
Nature Valley	4	30–40
Peanut: 1 bar / **Nature Valley**	5	30–40
Vegetarian meat substitutes		
(gluten base unless noted)		
Bologna: ½-in slice / **Loma Linda**	11	50–60
Burgers: 1 burger / **Loma Linda**		
Sizzle Burgers	10	50–60
Chicken: (4-in diam) ½-in slice /		
Loma Linda	10	50–60
Frankfurters: 1 frank / **Loma Linda**		
Big Franks	6	40–50
Linketts: 1 link / **Loma Linda**	3.5	40–50
Little Links: 1 link / **Loma Linda**	3	60–70
Meatballs: 1 ball / **Loma Linda**	1.7	30–40
Nuteena: ½-in slice / **Loma Linda**		
(peanut-butter base)	14	60–70
Proteena: ½-in slice / **Loma Linda**		
(gluten-peanut-butter base)	6	30–40
Redi-Burger: ½-in slice /		
Loma Linda	6	30–40

	FAT GRAMS	PERCENT OF CALORIES FROM FAT
Roast beef: ½-in slice / **Loma Linda**	12	50–60
Salami: ½-in slice / **Loma Linda**	12	50–60
Sausage: 1 link / **Loma Linda** Breakfast Links	2.3	40–50
Sausage: 1 piece / **Loma Linda** Breakfast Sausage	7.3	40–50
Stew Pac: 2 oz / **Loma Linda**	1	10–20
Swiss Steak: 1 steak / **Loma Linda**	7	40–50
Tender Bits: 1 bit / **Loma Linda**	.3	10–20
Tender Rounds: 1 round / **Loma Linda**	2	30–40
Turkey: ½-in slice / **Loma Linda**	11	50–60
Vegeburger: ½ cup / **Loma Linda**	1	0–10
Vegeburger, unsalted: ½ cup / **Loma Linda**	1	0–10
Vegelona: ½-in slice / **Loma Linda**	2	10–20

Soy Milk

Soyagen, all purpose: 1 cup prepared / **Loma Linda**	7	40–50
Soyagen, carob: 1 cup prepared / **Loma Linda**	7	40–50
Soyalac, concentrated: 6 fl oz prepared / **Loma Linda**	6.5	40–50
Soyalac, powder: 6 fl oz prepared / **Loma Linda**	6.5	40–50
I-Soyalac, concentrated: 6 fl oz prepared / **Loma Linda**	6.4	40–50

Herbs and Spices

Only trace amount of fat

Ice Cream and Similar Frozen Products

	FAT GRAMS	PERCENT OF CALORIES FROM FAT
½ cup unless noted		
Ice cream		
Black raspberry / **Breyers**	6	40–50
Black walnut / **Meadow Gold**	9	50–60
Butter almond / **Sealtest**	9	50–60
Butter almond, chocolate / **Breyers**	9	50–60
Butter brickle / **Sealtest**	7	40–50
Butter pecan / **Meadow Gold**	9	50–60
Butter pecan / **Sealtest**	10	50–60
Caramel pecan crunch / **Breyers**	8	40–50
Cherry Nugget / **Sealtest**	7	40–50
Cherry-vanilla / **Breyers**	7	40–50
Cherry-vanilla / **Meadow Gold**	6	30–40
Cherry-vanilla / **Sealtest**	6	40–50
Chocolate / **Breyers**	8	40–50
Chocolate / **Meadow Gold**	6	30–40
Chocolate / **Sealtest**	7	40–50
Chocolate / **Swift's**	6	40–50
Chocolate almond / **Breyers**	10	50–60
Chocolate almond / **Sealtest**	9	50–60
Chocolate chip / **Meadow Gold**	8	40–50
Chocolate chip / **Sealtest**	8	40–50

	FAT GRAMS	PERCENT OF CALORIES FROM FAT
Chocolate Revel / **Meadow Gold**	6	30–40
Coconut / **Sealtest**	9	50–60
Coffee / **Breyers**	8	50–60
Dutch chocolate almond / **Breyers**	10	50–60
Lemon / **Sealtest**	7	40–50
Maple walnut / **Sealtest**	9	50–60
Mint chocolate chip / **Breyers**	9	50–60
Peach / **Meadow Gold**	6	40–50
Peach / **Sealtest**	5	40–50
Pineapple / **Sealtest**	6	40–50
Southern pecan butterscotch / **Breyers**	9	50–60
Strawberry / **Breyers**	6	40–50
Strawberry / **Meadow Gold**	6	30–40
Strawberry / **Sealtest**	5.5	30–40
Strawberry / **Swift's**	6	40–50
Vanilla / **Breyers**	8	40–50
Vanilla / **Meadow Gold**	7	40–50
Vanilla / **Meadow Gold** Golden	7	40–50
Vanilla / **Sealtest**	7	40–50
Vanilla / **Swift's**	7	40–50
Vanilla, French / **Sealtest**	7	40–50
Vanilla-flavored cherry / **Sealtest** Royale	6	30–40
Vanilla-flavored red raspberry / **Sealtest** Royale	6	30–40
Vanilla fudge twirl / **Breyers**	8	40–50
Ice milk		
Banana-strawberry twirl / **Sealtest Light N' Lively**	2	10–20
Chocolate / **Sealtest Light N' Lively**	2	10–20
Chocolate / **Swift Light 'n Easy**	3	20–30
Coffee / **Sealtest Light N' Lively**	2	10–20
Fudge twirl / **Sealtest Light N' Lively**	2	10–20

	FAT GRAMS	PERCENT OF CALORIES FROM FAT
Neapolitan / Sealtest Light N' Lively	2	10–20
Peach / Sealtest Light N' Lively	2	10–20
Strawberry / Sealtest Light N' Lively	2	10–20
Strawberry / Swift's Light 'n Easy	3	20–30
Vanilla / Scaltest Light N' Lively	2	10–20
Vanilla / Swift Light 'n Easy	3	20–30
Sherbet		
Lemon / Sealtest	1	0–10
Lemon-Lime / Sealtest	1	0–10
Lime / Meadow Gold	1	0–10
Lime / Sealtest	1	0–10
Orange / Meadow Gold	1	0–10
Orange / Sealtest	1	0–10
Pineapple / Meadow Gold	1	0–10
Pineapple / Sealtest	1	0–10
Rainbow / Sealtest	1	0–10
Red raspberry / Sealtest	1	0–10
Strawberry / Sealtest	1	0–10

ICE CREAM BARS

1 bar or piece

Almond, toasted / Good Humor	14	50–60
Banana: 2½ fl oz bar / Fudgsicle	.1	0–10
Chocolate: 2½ fl oz bar / Bi-Sicle	2.1	10–20
Chocolate: 2½ fl oz bar / Fudgsicle	.3	0–10
Chocolate Eclair / Good Humor	13	50–60
Creamsicle: 2½ fl oz bar	2.6	30–40
Dreamsicle: 2½ fl oz bar	1.4	10–20
Ice Whammy, assorted flavors / Good Humor	0	0
Popsicle, all fruit flavors: 3 fl oz bar	0	0
Sandwich / Good Humor	6	20–30

	FAT GRAMS	PERCENT OF CALORIES FROM FAT
Strawberry shortcake / **Good Humor**	13	50–60
Whammy assorted ice cream / **Good Humor**	7	60–70
Whammy Chip Crunch / **Good Humor**	7	50–60
Vanilla, chocolate-coated / **Good Humor**	13	60–70

Italian Foods

See also Pizza and Spaghetti

	FAT GRAMS	PERCENT OF CALORIES FROM FAT
Cannelloni Florentine w veal, spinach, cheese and sauce, frozen: 13 oz / **Weight Watchers**	12	20–30
Eggplant Parmigiana, frozen: 4 oz / **Buitoni**	12.5	50–60
Eggplant Parmigiana, frozen: 13 oz / **Weight Watchers**	13	40–50
Lasagna		
Canned: 10 oz / **Hormel**	15	30–40
Canned: 7½ oz can / **Hormel** Short Orders	15	50–60
Frozen: 4 oz / **Buitoni** 26 oz	4.8	30–40
Frozen: 4 oz / **Buitoni** family size	6.6	30–40
Frozen w meat sauce: 4 oz / **Buitoni** 14 oz	5.8	30–40
Frozen: 7 oz / **Green Giant** Oven Bake Entrees	12	30–40

	FAT GRAMS	PERCENT OF CALORIES FROM FAT
Frozen: 9 oz / **Green Giant**		
Boil-in-Bag Entrees	11	30–40
Frozen: 10½ oz / **Stouffer's**	14	30–40
Frozen: 1 entree / **Swanson**		
Hungry-Man	28	40–50
Frozen w cheese, veal, sauce:		
13 oz / **Weight Watchers**	10	20–30
Mix, prepared 1/5 pkg /		
Golden Grain Stir-n Serv	3	10–20
Manicotti, frozen w sauce:		
4 oz / **Buitoni**	6.9	30–40
Manicotti, frozen wo sauce: 4 oz /		
Buitoni	7.9	30–40
Ravioli		
Beef in sauce, canned: 7½ oz /		
Franco-American	6	20–30
Beef in sauce, canned: 7½ oz /		
Franco-American Raviolos	6	20–30
Cheese, canned: ½ can / **Buitoni**	5	20–30
Cheese, frozen: 4 oz /		
Buitoni 12 Count Round	11.2	30–40
Cheese, frozen: 4 oz / **Buitoni**		
40 Count	12.4	30–40
Meat, canned: ½ can / **Buitoni**	8	30–40
Meat, frozen: 4 oz / **Buitoni**		
40 Count	7.2	10–20
Meat, frozen: 4 oz / **Buitoni**		
Raviolettes	4	10–20
Ravioli Parmigiana, meat, frozen:		
4 oz / **Buitoni**	9.7	40–50
Rotini, in tomato sauce, canned: 7½		
oz / **Franco-American**	4	10–20
Rotini and meatballs, in tomato sauce,		
canned: 7¼ oz /		
Franco-American	9	30–40

	FAT GRAMS	PERCENT OF CALORIES FROM FAT
Sausage and peppers w rigati, frozen:		
4 oz / **Buitoni**	10	50–60
Shells w sauce, frozen: 4 oz / **Buitoni**	1.4	0–10
Shrimp Marinara w shells, frozen:		
4 oz / **Buitoni**	1.6	10–20
Spaghetti w sauce and veal:		
1 entree / **Swanson "TV"**	15	40–50
Veal Parmigiana		
Frozen: 5 oz / **Banquet**		
Cookin' Bag	16.2	50–60
Frozen: 7 oz / **Green Giant**		
Oven Bake Entrees	17	40–50
Frozen w spaghetti twists: 4 oz /		
Buitoni	7	30–40
Frozen w tomato sauce: 32 oz /		
Banquet Buffet Supper	87.3	50–60
Frozen w zucchini: 9½ oz /		
Weight Watchers	9	30–40
Ziti, baked w sauce, frozen: 4 oz /		
Buitoni	.9	0–10
Ziti w veal and sauce, frozen:		
13 oz / **Weight Watchers**	8	10–20

Jams, Jellies, Preserves, Butters, Marmalade

Only traces of fat per tablespoon

Liqueurs and Brandies

No fat

Macaroni

	FAT GRAMS	PERCENT OF CALORIES FROM FAT
Plain: 1 cup cooked firm stage	.7	0–10
Plain: 1 cup cooked tender stage	.6	0–10
And beef, in tomato sauce, canned:		
7½ oz / **Franco-American**		
Beefy	8	30–40
And beef w tomato sauce, frozen: 9 oz /		
Green Giant Boil-in-Bag		
Entrees	8	30–40
And beef, frozen: 32 oz / **Banquet**		
Buffet Supper	40.9	30–40
And beef w tomatoes, frozen: ½ pkg /		
Stouffer's 11½ oz	8	30–40
And cheese		
Canned: 7¼ oz / **Franco-American**	7	30–40
Canned: 7¼ oz / **Hormel**		
Short Orders	6	10–20
Frozen: 8 oz / **Banquet**	10	30–40
Frozen: 32 oz / **Banquet**		
Buffet Supper	45.5	30–40
Frozen: 8 oz / **Banquet**		
Cookin' Bag	10.2	30–40
Frozen: 9 oz / **Green Giant**		
Boil-in-Bag Entrees	15	40–50
Frozen: 8 oz / **Green Giant**		
Oven Bake Entrees	13	40–50
Frozen: 10 oz / **Howard Johnson's**	32.4	50–60

	FAT GRAMS	PERCENT OF CALORIES FROM FAT
Frozen: 19 oz / **Howard Johnson's**	61.6	50–60
Frozen: 1 pkg / **Morton** Casserole	11	30–40
Frozen: ½ pkg / **Stouffer's** 12 oz	12	40–50
Frozen: 7 oz / **Swanson**	10	30–40
Mix, dry: 1.8 oz / **Ann Page**	2	0–10
Mix, prepared: ¼ pkg / **Betty Crocker**	14	40–50
Mix, prepared: 1 pouch / **Betty Crocker** Mug-O-Lunch	5	10–20
Mix, prepared: ¼ pkg / **Golden Grain** Macaroni and Cheddar	2	0–10
Mix, prepared: ¾ cup / **Kraft**	13	40–50
Mix, prepared: ½ cup / **Pennsylvania Dutch Brand**	4	20–30
And meatballs, in tomato sauce, canned: 7½ oz / **Franco-American** Meatball Mac	9	30–40

Mayonnaise

1 tbsp	FAT GRAMS	PERCENT OF CALORIES FROM FAT
Ann Page	11	100
Best	11	100
Hellmann's	11	100

	FAT GRAMS	PERCENT OF CALORIES FROM FAT
Kraft Real	11	100
Mrs. Filbert's Real	11	100
Nu Made	11	100
Piedmont	11	100
Sultana	11	100
Flavored / Durkee Famous Sauce	7	90–100
Imitation / Mrs. Filbert's	4	90–100
Imitation / Piedmont	5	90–100
Imitation / Weight Watchers	4	90–100
Miracle Whip / Kraft	7	90–100
w relish / Mrs. Filbert's Relish Spread	8	90–100

Meat

FRESH

	FAT GRAMS	PERCENT OF CALORIES FROM FAT
Lean means trimmed of all visible fat.		

Beef

Chuck
  Boneless for stew

	FAT GRAMS	PERCENT OF CALORIES FROM FAT
Lean w fat, cooked: 10.7 oz (yield from 1 lb)	72.7	60–70
Lean, cooked (braised or stewed): 10.7 oz (yield from 1 lb)	28.9	30–40

	FAT GRAMS	PERCENT OF CALORIES FROM FAT
Rib roast or chuck rib steak		
Choice grade		
Lean w fat, cooked: 3 oz	31.2	70–80
Lean, cooked: 3 oz	11.8	40–50
Arm and round bone roasts or steaks		
Choice grade		
Lean w fat, cooked: 3 oz piece	16.3	50–60
Lean, cooked: 3 oz piece	6	30–40
Good grade		
Lean w fat, cooked: 3 oz piece	12.4	50–60
Lean, cooked: 3 oz piece	4.4	20–30
Flank steak, choice grade		
100% lean, cooked: 3 oz piece	4.4	30–40
Ground beef		
Regular (21% fat)		
Patty, cooked (3″ diam, ⅝″ thick—2.9 oz)	16.6	60–70
Lean (10% fat)		
Patty, cooked (3″ diam, ⅝″ thick—3 oz)	9.6	40–50
Plate beef		
Lean w fat, cooked: 9.3 oz (yield from 1 lb w bone)	98.5	70–80
Lean, cooked: 6.5 oz (yield from 1 lb wo bone)	14.2	30–40
Rib roast, choice grade		
Lean w fat, cooked: 3 oz	33.5	70–80
Lean, cooked: 3 oz	11.4	40–50
Rump roast, choice grade		
Lean w fat, cooked: 3 oz	23.2	60–70
Lean, cooked: 3 oz	7.9	30–40
Rump roast, good grade		
Lean w fat, cooked: 3 oz	19.9	60–70
Lean, cooked: 3 oz	6	30–40

	FAT GRAMS	PERCENT OF CALORIES FROM FAT
Steaks		
Club, choice grade		
Lean w fat, cooked: 9.8 oz		
(yield from 1 lb w bone)	112.9	70–80
Lean, cooked: 5.7 oz (yield		
from 1 lb w bone)	20.9	40–50
Porterhouse, choice grade		
Lean w fat, cooked: 10.6 oz		
(yield from 1 lb w bone)	127	80–90
Lean, cooked: 6.1 oz (yield		
from 1 lb w bone)	18.1	40–50
Sirloin, wedge and round- bone,		
choice grade		
Lean w fat, cooked: 3 oz	27.2	70–80
Lean, cooked: 3 oz	6.5	30–40
Sirloin, double-bone, flat bone,		
choice grade		
Lean w fat, cooked: 3 oz	29.5	70–80
Lean, cooked: 3 oz	8.1	30–40
Beef fat: 3½ oz, cooked	78.1	90–100
Brains, all varieties, raw: 1 lb		
(beef, calf, hog, sheep)	39	60–70
Heart		
Beef, lean, cooked: 3½ oz	5.7	20–30
Beef, lean w visible fat, cooked:		
3½ oz	29	60–70
Calf, cooked: 3½ oz	9.1	30–40
Hog, cooked: 3½ oz	6.9	30–40
Lamb, cooked: 3½ oz	14.4	40–50
Kidneys		
Beef, raw: 3½ oz	6.7	40–50
Beef, cooked: 3½ oz	12	40–50
Lamb, raw: 3½ oz	3.3	20–30

	FAT GRAMS	PERCENT OF CALORIES FROM FAT
Lamb		
Leg		
Lean w fat, roasted: 3 oz	16.1	60–70
Lean, cooked: 3 oz	6	30–40
Loin chops		
Lean w fat, cooked: 3.4 oz (yield from 1 chop—3 per lb)	27.9	70–80
Lean, cooked: 2.3 oz (yield from 1 chop—3 per lb)	4.9	30–40
Rib chops		
Lean w fat, cooked: 3.1 oz (yield from 1 chop—3 per lb)	31.7	70–80
Lean, cooked: 2 oz (yield from 1 chop—3 per lb)	6	40–50
Shoulder		
Lean w fat, cooked: 3 oz	23.1	70–80
Lean, cooked: 3 oz	8.5	40–50
Liver		
Beef, raw: 3½ oz	3.8	20–30
Calf, raw: 3½ oz	4.7	20–30
Hog, raw: 3½ oz	3.7	20–30
Lamb, raw: 3½ oz	3.9	20–30
Pork		
Loin and loin chops		
Lean w fat, cooked: 3 oz	24.2	70–80
Lean, cooked: 3 oz	12.1	50–60
Boston butt		
Lean w fat, cooked: 3 oz	24.2	70–80
Lean, roasted: 3 oz	12.2	50–60
Picnic		
Lean w fat, cooked: 3 oz	25.9	70–80
Lean, cooked: 3 oz	8.3	40–50

	FAT GRAMS	PERCENT OF CALORIES FROM FAT
Spareribs		
Lean w fat, cooked (braised): 6.3 oz (yield from 1 lb)	70	70–80
Rabbit, domesticated, cooked, stewed: 3½ oz	10.1	40–50
Raccoon, roasted: 3½ oz	14.5	50–60
Sweetbreads		
Beef (yearlings)		
Braised: 3½ oz	23.2	60–70
Calf		
Braised: 3½ oz	3.2	10–20
Tongue		
Beef, medium fat, raw: 3½ oz	15	60–70

Veal

Chuck cuts and boneless veal for stew		
Lean w fat, cooked: 3 oz	10.9	40 50
Loin		
Lean w fat, cooked: 3 oz	11.4	50–60
Rib roast		
Lean w fat, roasted: 3 oz	14.4	50–60
Round with rump (roasts and leg cutlets		
Lean w fat, cooked: 3 oz	9.4	40–50

CANNED, CURED, PROCESSED

Bacon, cooked		
Hormel Black Label / 1 slice	2.7	60–70
Hormel Range Brand / 1 slice	4	90–100
Hormel Red Label / 1 slice	3.2	60–70
Oscar Mayer / 1 slice	3.5	70–80
Swift Lazy Maple / 1 slice	3.4	70–80

	FAT GRAMS	PERCENT OF CALORIES FROM FAT
Swift Premium / 1 slice	3.3	70–80
Canadian style: 1 slice / **Oscar Mayer**	2	40–50
Banquet loaf: 1 slice / **Eckrich** 8 oz pkg	6	70–80
Banquet loaf: 1 slice / **Eckrich** Beef Smorgas Pac	4.5	30–40
Bar-B-Q Loaf: 1 slice / **Oscar Mayer**	3	50–60
Beef, chopped: 1 slice / **Eckrich** Slender Sliced	1.4	30–40
Beef, corned, canned: 1 oz / **Safeway**	2	50–60
Beef, corned brisket, cooked: 3½ oz / **Swift** Premium for Oven Roasting	20	60–70
Beef, corned, chopped: 1 slice / **Eckrich** Slender Sliced	1.4	30–40
Beef, dried, chunked and formed: ¾ oz / **Swift Premium**	0	0–10
Beef, smoked, sliced: 1 oz / **Safeway**	2	50–60
Beef, smoked, sliced: 1 oz / **Safeway** Spicy	2	40–50
Beef steaks, breaded, frozen: 4 oz / **Hormel**	30	70–80
Bologna		
Eckrich 12 oz pkg / 1 slice	8.5	80–90
Eckrich 16 oz pkg / 1 slice	8.5	80–90
Eckrich Smorgas Pac / 1 slice	7.5	70–80
Eckrich thick-sliced / 1 slice (12 oz pkg)	14	70–80
Eckrich thick-sliced / 1 slice (16 oz pkg)	15	70–80
Hormel / 1 oz	7.5	70–80

	FAT GRAMS	PERCENT OF CALORIES FROM FAT
Swift Premium / 1 oz	8.5	70–80
Beef: 1 slice / Eckrich 8 oz pkg	8	70–80
Beef: 1 slice / Eckrich 12 oz pkg	8	70–80
Beef: 1 slice / Eckrich Beef Smorgas Pac	6	70–80
Beef: 1 slice / Oscar Mayer	6.5	80–90
Coarse ground: 1 oz / Hormel	6	70–80
Fine ground: 1 oz / Hormel	7.5	80–90
Garlic: 1 slice / Eckrich	8.5	80–90
Ring: 2 oz / Eckrich	18	80–90
Ring, garlic: 1 slice / Eckrich	8.5	80–90
Ring, pickled: 2 oz / Eckrich	17	80–90
Braunschweiger: 1 oz / Oscar Mayer	9	70–80
Breakfast Strips: 1 strip / Swift Sizzlean	4	70–80
Frankfurters: 1 frank		
Eckrich 12 oz pkg	11	80–90
Eckrich Jumbo	17	80–90
Eckrich Skinless 16 oz pkg	13	70–80
Hormel Wieners 12 oz pkg	9.5	80–90
Hormel Wieners 16 oz pkg	13	80–90
Hormel Range Brand Wranglers Smoked Franks	16	80–90
Oscar Mayer Wieners	13	80–90
Beef / Eckrich	13	70–80
Beef / Eckrich Jumbo	17	80–90
Beef / Hormel Wieners 12 oz pkg	9.5	80–90
Beef / Hormel Wieners 16 oz pkg	12	70–80
Beef / Hormel Wranglers Smoked Franks	12	60–70
Beef / Oscar Mayer	13	80–90
Frozen, batter-wrapped / Hormel Corn Dogs	13	50–60
Frozen, batter-wrapped / Hormel Tater Dogs	12	50–60

	FAT GRAMS	PERCENT OF CALORIES FROM FAT
Gourmet Loaf: 1 slice / **Eckrich**	1.5	30–40
Gourmet Loaf: 1 slice / **Eckrich**		
Beef Smorgas Pac	1	30–40
Ham, luncheon type		
Cooked: 1 slice / **Eckrich**	1	20–30
Cooked: 1 oz / **Hormel**	1	20–30
Cooked, smoked: 1 slice /		
Oscar Mayer	1.5	40–50
Cooked, sliced: 1 oz / **Safeway**	3	50–60
Chopped, smoked: 1 slice / **Eckrich**		
Slender Sliced	2	40–50
Chopped: 1 oz / **Hormel**	6	70–80
Chopped: 2 oz / **Hormel** 8 lb can	16	70–80
Chopped: 1 slice / **Oscar Mayer**	5	60–70
Ham, whole, canned		
Oscar Mayer Jubilee / 4 oz	5	30–40
Swift Premium / 3½ oz	15	60–70
Swift Premium Hostess / 3½ oz	6	30–40
Ham, whole, plastic or other wrap		
Hormel Bone-In / 6 oz	23	60–70
Hormel Cure 81 / 6 oz	18	50–60
Hormel Curemaster / 6 oz	8	30–40
Swift Premium Hostess / 3½ oz	7	40–50
Ham slice, smoked: 4 oz /		
Oscar Mayer Jubilee	5	30–40
Ham steaks: 1 slice / **Oscar Mayer**		
Jubilee	3	30–40
Ham patties: 1 patty / **Hormel**	18.5	80–90
Ham patties: 1 patty / **Swift**		
Premium Brown 'n Serve	24	80–90
Ham and cheese loaf: 1 slice /		
Oscar Mayer	6	70–80
Honey Loaf: 1 slice / **Eckrich**	2	40–50
Honey Loaf: 1 slice / **Eckrich**		
Smorgas Pac	2	40–50

	FAT GRAMS	PERCENT OF CALORIES FROM FAT
Honey Loaf: 1 slice / **Oscar Mayer**	1.5	30–40
Liver, beef, thin sliced: 2.6 oz / **Swift's** Tru Tender	5	30–40
Liver cheese: 1 slice / **Oscar Mayer**	10	80–90
Luncheon meat: 1 slice / **Oscar Mayer**	9	80–90
Luncheon meat, spiced: 1 oz / **Hormel**	6	60–70
Old fashioned loaf: 1 slice / **Eckrich**	6	70–80
Old fashioned loaf: 1 slice / **Eckrich** Smorgas Pac	6	70–80
Old fashioned loaf: 1 slice / **Oscar Mayer**	4.5	60–70
Olive loaf: 1 slice / **Oscar Mayer**	4.5	60–70
Pastrami, chopped: 1 slice / **Eckrich** Slender Sliced	2.1	40–50
Pastrami, sliced: 1 oz / **Safeway**	2	40–50
Pepperoni: 1 oz / **Swift**	13	70–80
Pepperoni, sliced: 1 oz / **Hormel**	13	80–90
Pickle loaf: 1 slice / **Eckrich** 8 oz pkg	7.5	70–80
Pickle loaf: 1 slice / **Eckrich** Smorgas Pac	7.5	70–80
Pickle loaf, beef: 1 slice / **Eckrich** Smorgas Pac	5.5	70–80
Pickle and pimento loaf: 1 slice / **Oscar Mayer**	4.5	60–70
Polish sausage: 1 link / **Eckrich** Polska Kielbasa Skinless	16	70–80
Polish sausage ring: 2 oz / **Eckrich** Polska Kielbasa	19	80–90
Polish sausage ring: 3 oz / **Hormel** Kolbase	21	70–80
Polish sausage, smoked beef: 1 oz / **Frito-Lay**	5.5	60–70
Pork loin, chipped, smoked: 1 slice / **Eckrich** Slender Sliced	2	30–40

	FAT GRAMS	PERCENT OF CALORIES FROM FAT
Pork steaks, breaded, frozen: 3 oz / **Hormel**	15	60–70
Salami		
Hormel Dairy Hard / 1 oz	10	70–80
Hormel Di Lusso Genoa / 1 oz	11	70–80
Oscar Mayer Beef Cotto / 1 slice	4	70–80
Oscar Mayer for Beer / 1 slice	4	70–80
Oscar Mayer Cotto / 1 slice	4	70–80
Oscar Mayer Hard / 1 slice	3.3	70–80
Swift Premium Genoa / 1 oz	10	70–80
Swift Premium Hard / 1 oz	9	70–80
Sausage, beef, smoked: 2 oz / **Eckrich**	19	80–90
Sausage, pork, smoked: 3 oz / **Hormel** No-Link	27	80–90
Sausage Links		
Hormel Brown 'n Serve / 1 sausage	7.2	80–90
Hormel Midget Links / 1 sausage	9.2	70–80
Hormel Little Sizzlers / 1 sausage	6	70–80
Oscar Mayer Little Friers / 1 link	5.5	70–80
Swift's The Original / 1 link	7	80–90
Swift Premium Brown 'n Serve Kountry Kured / 1 link	8	60–70
Swift Premium Bacon 'n Sausage / 1 link	6	70–80
Beef, cooked: 1 link / **Swift** Premium Brown 'n Serve	8	80–90
Sausage Links, smoked		
Eckrich 16 oz pkg / 1 link	17	80–90
Eckrich Skinless	10	70–80
Eckrich Smok-Y-Links / 1 link	6.5	70–80
Eckrich Skinless Smok-Y-Links / 1 link	7	70–80
Hormel Smokies / 1 sausage	8.2	70–80
Oscar Mayer / 1 link	12	70–80

	FAT GRAMS	PERCENT OF CALORIES FROM FAT
Beef: 1 link / **Eckrich**		
Smok-Y-Links	6	70–80
Spam: 3 oz / **Hormel**	23	70–80
Spam w cheese chunks: 3 oz / **Hormel**	22	70–80
Spam smoke-flavored: 3 oz / **Hormel**	24	80–90
Summer sausage: 1 slice / **Oscar Mayer**		
Thuringer Cervelat	6.4	80–90
Summer sausage, beef: 1 slice /		
Oscar Mayer	6	70–80
Summer sausage, beef: 1 oz /		
Swift Premium	8	70–80
Thuringer: 1 oz / **Hormel Old**		
Smokehouse	9	80–90
Veal steaks, frozen: 4 oz / **Hormel**	4	20–30
Veal steaks, frozen, breaded: 4 oz /		
Hormel	13	40–50
Vienna sausage, canned: 1 piece /		
Hormel	4.5	70–80

MEAT ENTREES, CANNED

	FAT GRAMS	PERCENT OF CALORIES FROM FAT
Beef w barbecue sauce: 5 oz /		
Morton House	11	40–50
Beef, dried, creamed: 7½ oz /		
Hormel Short Orders	10	50–60
Beef, goulash: 7½ oz can / **Hormel**		
Short Orders	12	40–50
Beef, sliced w gravy: 6¼ oz can /		
Morton House	12	50–60
Beef stew		
Dinty Moore / 7½ oz	9	40–50
Dinty Moore Short Orders /		
7½ oz can	8	40–50
Morton House / 8 oz	13	40–50
Swanson / 7½ oz	7	30–40

	FAT GRAMS	PERCENT OF CALORIES FROM FAT
Hash, beef w potatoes: 7½ oz can / **Dinty Moore Short Orders**	12	40–50
Hash, corned beef: 7½ oz / **Ann Page**	28	60–70
Hash, corned beef: 7½ oz / **Mary Kitchen**	26	50–60
Hash, corned beef: 7½ oz can / **Mary Kitchen Short Orders**	25	50–60
Hash, roast beef: 7½ oz / **Mary Kitchen**	27	60–70
Hash, roast beef: 7½ oz can / **Mary Kitchen Short Orders**	23	50–60
Pork, sliced w gravy: 6¼ oz / **Morton House**	12	50–60
Salisbury steak w mushroom gravy: 4 1 / 6 oz / **Morton House**	11	60–70
Sloppy Joe: 7½ oz can / **Hormel Short Orders**	22	50–60
Stew, meatball: 6¼ oz / **Morton House**	18	50–60
Stew Mulligan: 7½ oz can / **Dinty Moore Short Orders**	14	50–60

MEAT ENTREES, FROZEN

Beef, chipped, creamed: 5 oz / **Banquet** Cookin' Bag	4.1	20–30
Beef, chipped, creamed: 5½ oz pkg / **Stouffer's**	16	60–70
Beef, sliced: 1 entree / **Swanson** Hungry-Man	9	20–30
Beef, sliced w barbecue sauce: 5 oz / **Banquet** Cookin' Bag	2.6	10–20

	FAT GRAMS	PERCENT OF CALORIES FROM FAT
Beef, sliced w gravy: 32 oz / **Banquet** Buffet Supper	41.8	40–50
Beef, sliced w gravy: 5 oz / **Banquet** Cookin' Bag	4.3	30–40
Beef, sliced w gravy: 5 oz / **Green Giant** Boil-in-Bag Toast Toppers	4	20–30
Beef, sliced w gravy and whipped potatoes: 1 entree / **Swanson** "TV"	7	30–40
Beef Stroganoff: 9¾ oz pkg / **Stouffer's**	20	50–60
Green pepper steak: 10½ oz pkg / **Stouffer's**	13	30–40
Meat Loaf		
Banquet Buffet Supper / 32 oz	108.2	60–70
Banquet Cookin' Bag / 5 oz	15.6	60–70
Banquet Man-Pleaser / 19 oz	57.7	50–60
Morton Country Table / 1 entree	20	40–50
w tomato sauce and whipped potatoes: 1 entree / **Swanson** "TV"	16	40–50
Meatballs w gravy and whipped potatoes: 1 entree / **Swanson** "TV"	17	40–50
Noodles and beef: 32 oz / **Banquet** Buffet Supper	26.4	30–40
Salisbury Steak		
Banquet Man-Pleaser / 19 oz	48	40–50
Morton Country Table / 1 entree	24	40–50
Stouffer's 12 oz / ½ pkg	15	50–60
Swanson Hungry-Man / 1 entree	39	50–60
w crinkle-cut potatoes: 1 entree / **Swanson** "TV"	22	50–60

	FAT GRAMS	PERCENT OF CALORIES FROM FAT
w gravy: 32 oz / **Banquet** Buffet Supper	109.1	60–70
w gravy: 5 oz / **Banquet** Cookin' Bag	18.5	60–70
w gravy: 7 oz / **Green Giant** Oven Bake Entrees	18	50–60
w tomato sauce: 9 oz / **Green Giant** Boil-in-Bag Entrees	25	50–60
Sausage, cheese and tomato pies: 7 oz / **Weight Watchers**	13	30–40
Sloppy Joe: 5 oz / **Banquet** Cookin' Bag	12.4	50–60
Sloppy Joe: 5 oz / **Green Giant** Boil-in-Bag Toast Toppers	6	30–40
Stew, beef: 32 oz / **Banquet** Buffet Supper	14.5	10–20
Stew, beef: 9 oz / **Green Giant** Boil-in-Bag Entrees	3	10–20
Stew, beef: 1 pkg / **Stouffer's** 10 oz	17	40–50
Stew, beef w biscuits: 7 oz / **Green Giant** Oven Bake Entrees	6	20–30
Stuffed cabbage w beef, in tomato sauce: 7 oz / **Green Giant** Oven Bake Entrees	12	40–50
Stuffed green peppers w beef: 7 oz / **Green Giant** Oven Bake Entrees	11	40–50

MEAT SUBSTITUTES

Breakfast Links: 1 link / **Morningstar Farms**	4.5	60–70
Breakfast Patties: 1 pattie / **Morningstar Farms**	7.2	50–60
Breakfast Strips: 1 strip / **Morningstar Farms**	3.7	80–90

	FAT GRAMS	PERCENT OF CALORIES FROM FAT
Grillers: one griller / **Morningstar Farms**	13.5	50–60
Luncheon slices: 1 slice / **Morningstar Farms**	.8	20–30

Mexican Foods

	FAT GRAMS	PERCENT OF CALORIES FROM FAT
Beans, refried, canned: ½ cup / **Ortega** Lightly Spicy	4	20–30
Beans, refried, canned: ½ cup / **Ortega** True Bean	4	20–30
Burritos, beef, canned: 4 oz / **Hormel**	8	30–40
Chiles, diced, canned: 1 oz / **Ortega**	.1	0–10
Chiles, in strips, canned: 1 oz / **Ortega**	0	0–10
Chiles, whole, canned: 1 oz / **Ortega**	0	0–10
Chili con carne, canned		
w beans: 8 oz / **A & P**	30	60–70
w beans: 7½ oz / **Hormel**	18	50–60
Hormel Short Orders	16	40–50
w beans: 7½ oz / **Morton House**	18	40–50
w beans: 7¾ oz / **Swanson**	15	40–50
w beans, low sodium: 7¾ oz / **Campbell**	16	40–50
wo beans: 7½ oz / **Hormel**	26	60–70
wo beans: 7½ oz / **Morton House**	20	50–60

	FAT GRAMS	PERCENT OF CALORIES FROM FAT
Chili Mac, canned: 7½ oz / **Hormel Short Orders**	10	40–50
Enchiladas		
Frozen: 1 dinner / **El Chico**	37	30–40
Frozen, beef w cheese and chili gravy: 32 oz / **Banquet** Buffet Supper	54.5	40–50
Frozen, beef and cheese w gravy: 3 enchiladas / **El Chico**	30	30–40
Frozen, beef w gravy: 3 enchiladas / **El Chico**	33	40–50
Frozen, beef w sauce: 6 oz / **Banquet** Cookin' Bag	6.6	20–30
Queso dinner, frozen: 1 dinner / **El Chico**	20	20–30
Peppers, hot, diced, or whole, canned: 1 oz / **Ortega**	.1	0–10
Salsa, green chile, canned: 1 oz / **Ortega**	0	0–10
Saltillo dinner, frozen: 1 dinner / **El Chico**	30	20–30
Taco shell: 1 shell / **Ortega**	1.9	30–40
Tacos, beef, frozen: 3 tacos / **El Chico**	17	30–40
Tacos, prepared: 1 taco / **Ortega**	12	40–50
Tamales, beef, canned: 1 tamale / **Hormel**	5.5	70–80
Tamales, beef, in jar: 2 tamales / **Swift Derby**	18	60–70
Tomatoes and hot green chiles, canned: 1 oz / **Ortega**	0	0–10
Tortilla, corn: 1 (6½" diameter)	.4	0–10

Milk

	FAT GRAMS	PERCENT OF CALORIES FROM FAT
1 cup unless noted		
Milk, whole	8.1	40–50
Lowfat milk (2% fat)	4.7	30–40
Lowfat milk (1% fat)	2.6	20–30
Skim milk	.4	0–10
Chocolate milk	8.5	30–40
Lowfat chocolate (2% fat)	5	20–30
Lowfat chocolate (1% fat)	2.5	10–20
Sweetened condensed whole milk	26.6	20–30
Evaporated whole milk	19	50–60
Evaporated skim milk	.5	0–10
Dried whole milk	34.2	40–50
Nonfat dry milk, instant: 1⅓ cups	.7	0–10
Nonfat dry milk, regular	.9	0–10
Dried buttermilk, sweet cream	6.9	10–20
Buttermilk, cultured (skim milk)	2.2	10–20
Goat milk	9.8	50–60
Human milk	9.6	70–80

FLAVORED MILK BEVERAGES

All flavors, canned: 10 fl oz / **Carnation** Slender	5	20–30
All flavors, mix: 1 env prepared / **Lucerne** Instant Breakfast	9	20–30
Chocolate mixes		
Carnation Instant Breakfast / 1 env	1	0–10

	FAT GRAMS	PERCENT OF CALORIES FROM FAT
Carnation Slender / 1 env	1	0–10
Ovaltine / ¾ oz	1	10–20
PDQ / 3½ tsp	.3	0–10
Safeway / 2 tsp dry w 8 fl oz whole milk	8	30–40
mix prepared: 1 pouch / **Pillsbury** Instant Breakfast	9	20–30
Dutch, mix: 1 env / **Carnation** Slender	1	0–10
Malt, mix: 1 env / **Carnation** Instant Breakfast	1	0–10
Malt, mix: 1 env / **Carnation** Slender	1	0–10
Malt, mix, prepared: 1 pouch / **Pillsbury** Instant Breakfast	9	20–30
Coffee, mix: 1 env / **Carnation** Instant Breakfast	0	0
Coffee, mix: 1 env / **Carnation** Slender	0	0
Eggnog, mix: 1 env / **Carnation** Instant Breakfast	0	0
Eggnog, mix: 2 heaping tbsp / **PDQ**	.5	0–10
Malt-flavored, instant: 3 heaping tsp / **Carnation**	1.7	10–20
Malt-flavored, chocolate, instant: 3 heaping tsp / **Carnation**	1	10–20
Malt-flavor, mix: ¾ oz / **Ovaltine**	1	10–20
Strawberry, mix: 1 env / **Carnation** Instant Breakfast	0	0–10
Strawberry, mix: 3½ tsp / **PDQ**	0	0–10
Strawberry, mix, prepared: 1 pouch / **Pillsbury** Instant Breakfast	9	20–30
Strawberry, wild, mix: 1 env / **Carnation** Slender	0	0
Vanilla, mix: 1 env / **Carnation** Instant Breakfast	0	0

	FAT GRAMS	PERCENT OF CALORIES FROM FAT
Vanilla, mix prepared: 1 pouch / **Pillsbury** Instant Breakfast	0	20–30
Vanilla, French, mix: 1 env / **Carnation** Slender	0	0

Muffins: English and Sweet

	FAT GRAMS	PERCENT OF CALORIES FROM FAT
1 muffin unless noted		
Apple cinnamon, mix, prepared / **Betty Crocker**	5	20–30
Apple cinnamon, refrigerator, to bake / **Pillsbury**	5	30–40
Banana nut, mix, prepared / **Betty Crocker** Chiquita	7	30–40
Blueberry		
Thomas' Toast-R-Cakes	4	30–40
Frozen / **Howard Johnson's** Toasties	4.9	30–40
Frozen / **Morton**	3	20–30
Frozen / **Morton** Rounds	3	20–30
Frozen / **Pepperidge Farm**	4	20–30
Mix, prepared / **Betty Crocker**	4	20–30

	FAT GRAMS	PERCENT OF CALORIES FROM FAT
Bran / **Oroweat** Bran'nola	1	0–10
Bran / **Thomas'** Toast-R-Cakes	3	20–30
Corn		
Thomas'	8	30–40
Thomas' Toast-R-Cakes	4	30–40
Frozen / **Howard Johnson's** Toasties	3.4	20–30
Frozen / **Morton**	4	20–30
Frozen / **Morton** Rounds	4	20–30
Frozen / **Pepperidge Farm**	5	30–40
Frozen / **Thomas'** Toast-R-Cakes	4	30–40
Mix, prepared / **Betty Crocker**	5	20–30
Mix, prepared / **Flako**	4	20–30
Refrigerator, to bake / **Pillsbury**	5	30–40
English		
Arnold	1	0–10
Pepperidge Farm	1	0–10
Thomas'	1	0–10
Wonder	1	0–10
Frozen / **Thomas'**	1	0–10
Cinnamon-raisin / **Pepperidge Farm**	1	0–10
Onion / **Thomas'**	1	0–10
Sourdough / **Oroweat**	1	0–10
Wheat / **Home Pride**	2	10–20
Honeyberry wheat / **Oroweat**	1	0–10
Honey Butter / **Oroweat**	1	0–10
Orange, frozen / **Howard Johnson's** Toasties	5.4	40–50
Orange, mix, prepared / **Betty Crocker** Sunkist	5	20–30
Pineapple, mix, prepared / **Betty Crocker**	3	20–30
Raisin / **Oroweat**	1	0–10
Raisin / **Wonder** Rounds	3	10–20

	FAT GRAMS	PERCENT OF CALORIES FROM FAT
Raisin bran, frozen / **Pepperidge Farm**	5	30–40
Sourdough / **Wonder**	1	0–10
Wild blueberry, mix, prepared / **Duncan Hines**	3	20–30

Noodles and Noodle Dishes

	FAT GRAMS	PERCENT OF CALORIES FROM FAT
Noodles, plain, cooked: 1 cup	2.4	0–10
Almondine, mix, prepared: ¼ pkg / **Betty Crocker**	12	40–50
w beef: 7½ oz can / **Hormel Short Orders**	14	50–60
w beef-flavored sauce, mix, prepared: 1 pouch / **Betty Crocker** Mug-O-Lunch	3	10–20
w beef sauce, mix, prepared: ½ cup / **Pennsylvania Dutch Brand**	1	0–10
w butter sauce, mix, prepared: ½ cup / **Pennsylvania Dutch Brand**	4	20–30
w cheese, mix, prepared: 1/5 pkg / **Noodle-Roni** Parmesano	2	10–20
w cheese sauce, mix, prepared: ½ cup / **Pennsylvania Dutch Brand**	3	10–20
w chicken, canned: 7½ oz / **Dinty Moore**	12	40–50
w chicken sauce, mix, prepared: ½ cup / **Pennsylvania Dutch Brand**	3	10–20
Romanoff, frozen: ⅓ pkg / **Stouffer's**	9	40–50

	FAT GRAMS	PERCENT OF CALORIES FROM FAT
Romanoff, mix, prepared: ¼ pkg / **Betty Crocker**	12	40–50
Stroganoff mix: 2 oz / **Pennsylvania Dutch Brand**	3	10–20
Stroganoff, mix, prepared: ¼ pkg / **Betty Crocker**	11	40–50
w tuna, frozen: ½ pkg / **Stouffer's** 11½ oz	9	30–40

Nuts

SALTED AND FLAVORED

	FAT GRAMS	PERCENT OF CALORIES FROM FAT
1 oz unless noted (1 oz = about 1/5 cup)		
Almonds, dry roasted / **Planters**	15	70–80
Cashews		
Frito-Lay	14.1	70–80
Planters	14	70–80
Planters, unsalted	13	70–80
Dry roasted, jar / **A & P**	13	60–70
Dry roasted / **Planters**	13	70–80
Dry roasted / **Skippy**	13.3	70–80
Mixed		
Excel	16	70–80
w peanuts / **Planters**	16	80–90
wo peanuts / **A & P** Fancy	17	80–90
wo peanuts / **Planters**	17	80–90
Unsalted / **Planters**	15	70–80

	FAT GRAMS	PERCENT OF CALORIES FROM FAT
Dry roasted / **A & P**	14	70–80
Dry roasted / **Planters**	14	70–80
Dry roasted / **Skippy**	15.1	70–80
Peanuts		
A & P	15	70–80
Frito Lay	15.2	70–80
Planters Old Fashioned	15	70–80
Unsalted / **Planters**	15	70–80
Cocktail / **Planters**	15	70–80
Cocktail halves / **Excel**	15	70–80
Dry roasted, jar / **A & P**	14	70–80
Dry roasted / **Planters**	14	70–80
Dry roasted / **Skippy**	14.5	70–80
In the shell: 1 oz edible portion / **A & P**	14	70–80
In the shell: 1 oz edible portion / **A & P** Raw Fancies	14	70–80
In the shell: 1 oz edible portion / **Frito-Lay**	13.8	70–80
Spanish / **A & P**	15	70–80
Spanish / **Frito-Lay**	14.5	70–80
Spanish / **Planters**	15	70–80
Spanish, dry roasted / **Planters**	14	70–80
Virginia redskin / **Planters**	15	70–80
Pecans (pieces and chopped) / **A & P**	20	90–100
Pecans, dry roasted / **Planters**	19	90–100
Pistachios: 1 oz of edible portion / **Frito-Lay**	16.3	80–90
Pistachios, dry roasted / **Planters** Natural	15	80–90
Sesame Nut Mix / **Planters**	13	70–80
Tavern / **Planters**	15	70–80

UNFLAVORED, UNSALTED

Almonds		
Dried, in shell: 10 nuts	5.4	80–90

	FAT GRAMS	PERCENT OF CALORIES FROM FAT
Dried, in shell: 1 cup	16.9	80–90
Dried, shelled, chopped: 1 cup	70.5	80–90
Dried, shelled, chopped: 1 tbsp	4.3	80–90
Dried, shelled, slivered: 1 cup	62.3	80–90
Dried, shelled, whole: 1 cup	77	80–90
Roasted in oil: 1 cup	90.6	80–90
Beechnuts, in shell: 1 lb	138.4	70–80
Beechnuts, shelled: 1 lb	226.8	70–80
Brazil nuts, in shell: 1 cup	39.2	90–100
Brazil nuts, shelled: 1 cup	93.7	90–100
Brazil nuts, shelled: 1 oz or 6-8 kernels	19	90–100
Butternuts, in shell: 1 lb	38.9	80–90
Butternuts, shelled: 1 lb	277.6	80–90
Cashew nuts, roasted in oil: 1 cup	64	70–80
Cashew nuts, roasted in oil: 1 lb	207.3	70–80
Chestnuts, fresh, in shell: 1 cup	1.5	0–10
Chestnuts, fresh, in shell: 1 lb	5.5	0–10
Chestnuts, fresh, shelled: 1 cup	2.4	0–10
Chestnuts, fresh, shelled: 1 lb	6.8	0–10
Filberts, in shell: 1 lb	130	80–90
Filberts, shelled, chopped: 1 cup	71.8	80–90
Filberts, shelled, whole: 1 cup	84.2	80–90
Peanuts		
Roasted in shell: 10 jumbo nuts	8.8	70–80
Roasted in shell: 1 lb	148	70–80
Roasted (Spanish and Virginia) chopped: 1 cup	71.7	70–80
Roasted (Spanish and Virginia): 1 lb	117.9	70–80
Pecans		
In shell: 10 oversize (55 or fewer per lb)	31	90–100
In shell: 10 extra large (56-63 per lb)	28.7	90–100

	FAT GRAMS	PERCENT OF CALORIES FROM FAT
In shell: 10 large		
(64-77 per lb)	24.5	90–100
Chopped or pieces: 1 cup	84	90–100
Chopped or pieces: 1 tbsp	5.3	90–100
Halves: 10 large	6.5	90–100
Halves: 10 jumbo	10	90–100
Halves: 10 mammoth	12.8	90–100
Pinenuts, Pignolias, shelled: 1 oz	13.4	70–80
Pinenuts, Pinon, shelled: 1 oz	17.2	70–80
Pistachio nuts, in shell: 1 lb	121.8	80–90
Pistachio nuts, shelled: 1 lb	243.6	80–90
Walnuts		
Black in shell: 1 lb	59.2	80–90
Black, shelled, chopped or broken kernels		
1 cup	74.1	80–90
1 tbsp	4.7	80–90
Persian or English, in shell: 1 lb	130.6	80–90
Persian or English, shelled, halves:		
1 cup	64	80–90
Persian or English, chopped:		
1 tbsp	5.1	80–90
Persian or English: 10 large nuts	31.7	80–90

O_{ils}

All kinds of oils (corn, cottonseed, safflower, sesame, soybean, peanut, olive) have 216 fat grams per cup or 14 per tablespoon. About 100 percent of the calories from oils come from fat.

Olives

1 olive	FAT GRAMS	PERCENT OF CALORIES FROM FAT
Green, small	.4	90–100
Green, large	.5	90–100
Green, giant	.8	90–100
Ripe, black		
Ascolano, extra large	.6	90–100
Ascolano, giant	1	90–100
Ascolano, jumbo	1.1	90–100
Manzanillo, small	.4	90–100
Manzanillo, medium	.5	90–100
Manzanillo, large	.6	90–100
Manzanillo, extra large	.7	90–100
Mission, small	.6	90–100
Mission, medium	.7	90–100

	FAT GRAMS	PERCENT OF CALORIES FROM FAT
Mission, large	.8	90–100
Mission, extra large	1	90–100
Sevillano, giant	.7	90–100
Sevillano, jumbo	.8	90–100
Sevillano, colossal	1	90–100
Sevillano, supercolossal	1.2	90–100
Greek style, medium	.7	90–100
Greek style, extra large	1	90–100

Pancakes, Waffles and Similar Breakfast Foods

	FAT GRAMS	PERCENT OF CALORIES FROM FAT
Breakfast, frozen, French toast w sausages: 1 entree / **Swanson "TV"**	17	50–60
Breakfast, frozen, pancakes and sausages: 1 entree / **Swanson "TV"**	25	40–50
Breakfast, frozen, scrambled eggs w sausage and coffee cake: 1 entree / **Swanson "TV"**	31	50–60
Breakfast bars, chocolate chip: 1 bar / **Carnation**	10	40–50
Breakfast bars, chocolate crunch: 1 bar / **Carnation**	10	40–50
Breakfast bars, peanut butter crunch: 1 bar / **Carnation**	10	40–50
Breakfast squares: 1 bar / **General Mills**	8.5	30–40
Crepes, mix, prepared: 2 crepes 6-in diam / **Aunt Jemima**	4	30–40
French toast, frozen: 1 slice / **Downyflake**	7	40–50
French toast, frozen: 1 slice / **Aunt Jemima**	2.5	20–30

	FAT GRAMS	PERCENT OF CALORIES FROM FAT
French toast w cinnamon, frozen: 1 slice / **Aunt Jemima** Cinnamon Swirl	3.5	20–30
Fritters, apple, frozen: 1 fritter / **Mrs. Paul's**	6	40–50
Fritters, corn, frozen: 1 fritter / **Mrs. Paul's**	6	40–50
Pancakes, frozen: 1 pancake / **Downyflake**	3.5	30–40
Pancake batter, frozen: 3 cakes 4-in diam / **Aunt Jemima**	3	10–20
Pancake batter, frozen: 3 cakes 4-in diam / **Aunt Jemima** Blueberry	3	10–20
Pancake batter, frozen: 3 cakes 4-in diam / **Aunt Jemima** Buttermilk	2	10–20
Pancake, mix, prepared: 3 cakes 4-in diam		
Hungry Jack Complete	3	10–20
Hungry Jack Extra Lights	6	30–40
Tillie Lewis	1	0–10
Blueberry / **Hungry Jack**	16	40–50
Buttermilk / **Betty Crocker**	9	30–40
Buttermilk / **Betty Crocker** Complete	3	10–20
Buttermilk / **Hungry Jack**	11	40–50
Buttermilk / **Hungry Jack** Complete	3	10–20
Pancake-waffle mix prepared: 3 cakes 4-in diam		
Aunt Jemima Complete	3	10–20
Aunt Jemima Original	8	30–40
Log Cabin Complete	3	10–20
Log Cabin Regular	6	30–40
Buckwheat / **Aunt Jemima**	8	30–40
Buttermilk / **Aunt Jemima**	11	30–40

	FAT GRAMS	PERCENT OF CALORIES FROM FAT
Buttermilk / **Aunt Jemima**		
Complete	3	10–20
Buttermilk / **Log Cabin**	7	20–30
Whole wheat / **Aunt Jemima**	9	30–40
Waffles, frozen: 1 waffle		
Aunt Jemima Jumbo Original	3	30–40
Downyflake	1.5	20–30
Downyflake Hot 'n Buttery	2.5	30–40
Downyflake Jumbo	2	20–30
Eggo	5	30–40
Blueberry / **Aunt Jemima** Jumbo	3	30–40
Blueberry / **Downyflake**	2	20–30
Blueberry / **Eggo**	5	30–40
Bran / **Downyflake**	1.5	20–30
Bran / **Eggo**	8	40–50
Buttermilk / **Aunt Jemima** Jumbo	3	30–40
Buttermilk / **Downyflake**	2	20–30
Buttermilk / **Downyflake** Round	2.5	20–30
Strawberry / **Eggo**	5	30–40

Pastry

	FAT GRAMS	PERCENT OF CALORIES FROM FAT
Donuts, frozen: 1 donut		
Morton Mini	6	40–50
Bavarian creme / **Morton**	9	40–50
Boston creme / **Morton**	9	30–40
Chocolate iced / **Morton**	7	40–50
Glazed / **Morton**	7	40–50

	FAT GRAMS	PERCENT OF CALORIES FROM FAT
Jelly / **Morton**	8	40–50
Dumplings, apple, frozen:		
1 dumpling / **Pepperidge Farm**	17	50–60
Pie-Tarts, frozen: 1 tart		
Apple / **Pepperidge Farm**	16	50–60
Blueberry / **Pepperidge Farm**	15	50–60
Cherry / **Pepperidge Farm**	15	50–60
Lemon / **Pepperidge Farm**	19	50–60
Raspberry / **Pepperidge Farm**	19	50–60
Strudel, apple, frozen: 3 oz /		
Pepperidge Farm	13	40–50
Turnovers: 1 turnover		
Apple, frozen / **Pepperidge Farm**	21	50–60
Apple, refrigerator / **Pillsberry**	9	40–50
Blueberry, frozen /		
Pepperidge Farm	20	50–60
Blueberry, refrigerator / **Pillsbury**	9	40–50
Cherry, frozen / **Pepperidge Farm**	20	50–60
Cherry, refrigerator / **Pillsbury**	9	40–50
Peach, frozen / **Pepperidge Farm**	20	50–60
Raspberry, frozen /		
Pepperidge Farm	20	50–60

TOASTER PASTRIES

1 portion

Frosted, cinnamon brown sugar /		
Town House	5	20–30
Pop-Tart, blueberry / **Kellogg's**	6	20–30
Pop-Tart, brown sugar-cinnamon /		
Kellogg's	7	30–40
Pop-Tart, cherry / **Kellogg's**	6	20–30
Pop-Tart, concord grape / **Kellogg's**	6	20–30
Pop-Tart, raspberry / **Kellogg's**	6	20–30
Pop-Tart, strawberry / **Kellogg's**	6	20–30

	FAT GRAMS	PERCENT OF CALORIES FROM FAT
Pop-Tart, frosted, blueberry / **Kellogg's**	5	20–30
Pop-Tart, frosted, brown sugar-cinnamon / **Kellogg's**	7	30–40
Pop Tart, frosted, cherry / **Kellogg's**	6	20–30
Pop-Tart, frosted, chocolate fudge / **Kellogg's**	6	20–30
Pop-Tart, frosted, chocolate-peppermint / **Kellogg's**	6	20–30
Pop-Tart, frosted, chocolate vanilla creme / **Kellogg's**	7	30–40
Pop-Tart, frosted, concord grape / **Kellogg's**	5	20–30
Pop-Tart, frosted, dutch apple / **Kellogg's**	6	20–30
Pop-Tart, frosted, raspberry / **Kellogg's**	6	20–30
Pop-Tart, frosted, strawberry / **Kellogg's**	6	20–30

Pickles and Relishes

Trace amounts of fat

Pies

FROZEN

	FAT GRAMS	PERCENT OF CALORIES FROM FAT
1 whole pie		
Apple		
Banquet 20 oz	58.4	30–40
Morton 24 oz	78	30–40
Morton Mini 8 oz	25	30–40
Mrs. Smith's 8 in	90	40–50
Mrs. Smith's (natural juice) 8 in	138	40–50
Sara Lee	127.2	40–50
Dutch / **Mrs. Smith's** 8 in	78	30–40
Dutch / **Sara Lee**	75	30–40
Tart / **Mrs. Smith's** 8 in	54	30–40
Banana cream / **Banquet** 14 oz	57.6	40–50
Banana cream / **Morton** 16 oz	60	50–60
Banana cream / **Morton** Mini 3.5 oz	14	50–60
Banana cream / **Mrs. Smith's** Light 13.8	72	40–50
Banana cream / **Mrs. Smith's** 8 in	66	40–50
Blueberry		
Banquet 20 oz	60.7	30–40
Morton 24 oz	84	40–50
Morton Mini 8 oz	25	30–40
Mrs. Smith's 8 in	84	40–50
Mrs. Smith (natural juice) 8 in	102	40–50
Mrs. Smith's (natural juice) 9 in	138	40–50
Sara Lee	111.6	40–50
Boston cream / **Mrs. Smith's** 8 in	78	30–40
Cherry		
Banquet 20 oz	54.4	30–40
Morton 24 oz	84	40–50

	FAT GRAMS	PERCENT OF CALORIES FROM FAT
Morton Mini 8 oz	25	30–40
Mrs. Smith's 8 in	84	40–50
Mrs. Smith's (natural juice) 8 in	96	40–50
Mrs. Smith's (natural juice) 9 in	138	40–50
Sara Lee	102	40–50
Chocolate / **Mrs. Smith's** Light 13.8 oz	72	40–50
Chocolate cream / **Banquet** 14 oz	54.6	40–50
Chocolate cream / **Morton** 16 oz	72	50–60
Chocolate cream / **Morton** Mini 3.5 oz	16	50–60
Chocolate cream / **Mrs. Smith's** 8 in	72	40–50
Coconut / **Mrs. Smith's** Light 13.8 oz.	72	40–50
Coconut cream / **Banquet** 14 oz	61.3	50–60
Coconut cream / **Morton** 16 oz	66	50–60
Coconut cream / **Morton** Mini 3.5 oz	15	50–60
Coconut cream / **Mrs. Smith's** 8 in	66	40–50
Coconut custard / **Banquet** 20 oz	47.1	30–40
Coconut custard / **Morton** Mini 6.5 oz	15	30–40
Coconut custard / **Mrs. Smith's** 8 in	72	40–50
Custard / **Banquet** 20 oz	39.7	20–30
Egg custard / **Mrs. Smith's** 8 in	60	30–40
Lemon / **Mrs. Smith's** 8 in	102	40–50
Lemon cream / **Banquet** 14 oz	50.6	40–50
Lemon cream / **Morton** 16 oz	60	50–60
Lemon cream / **Morton** Mini 3.5 oz	14	50–60
Lemon cream / **Mrs. Smith's** 8 in	66	40–50
Lemon Krunch / **Mrs. Smith's** 8 in	96	30–40
Lemon meringue / **Mrs. Smith's** 8 in	60	30–40
Lemon yogurt / **Mrs. Smith's** 15.6 oz	54	30–40
Mince / **Morton** 24 oz	84	40–50
Mince / **Morton** Mini 8 oz	25	30–40
Mince / **Mrs. Smith's** 8 in	84	30–40
Mincemeat / **Banquet** 20 oz	57.3	30–40
Neopolitan cream / **Morton** 16 oz	66	50–60

	FAT GRAMS	PERCENT OF CALORIES FROM FAT
Neopolitan cream / **Mrs. Smith's** 8 in	72	40–50
Peach / **Banquet** 20 oz	59	30–40
Peach / **Morton** 24 oz	78	40–50
Peach / **Morton** Mini 8 oz	25	40–50
Peach / **Mrs. Smith's** 8 in	84	40–50
Peach (natural juice) / **Mrs. Smith's** 8 in	96	40–50
Peach (natural juice) / **Mrs. Smith's** 9 in	138	40–50
Peach / **Sara Lee**	109	40–50
Pecan / **Morton** Mini 6.5 oz	28	40–50
Pecan / **Mrs. Smith's** 8 in	120	40–50
Pineapple / **Mrs. Smith's** 8 in	84	40–50
Pineapple cheese / **Mrs. Smith's** 8 in	66	30–40
Pumpkin / **Banquet** 20 oz	41.1	20–30
Pumpkin / **Morton** 24 oz	48	30–40
Pumpkin / **Morton** Mini 8 oz	14	30–40
Pumpkin / **Mrs. Smith's** 8 in	60	30–40
Raisin / **Mrs. Smith's** 8 in	84	40–50
Strawberry cream / **Banquet** 14 oz	49.3	40–50
Strawberry cream / **Morton** 16 oz	60	50–60
Strawberry cream / **Mrs. Smith's** 8 in	66	40–50
Strawberry-rhubarb / **Mrs Smith's** 8 in	84	40–50
Strawberry-rhubarb (natural juice) / **Mrs. Smith's** 8 in	96	40–50
Strawberry-rhubarb (natural juice) / **Mrs. Smith's** 9 in	138	40–50
Strawberry yogurt / **Mrs. Smith's** 15.6 oz	60	40–50

PIE MIXES

Prepared: 1 whole pie

Boston cream / **Betty Crocker**	48	20–30
Chocolate cream / **Pillsbury** No Bake	114	40–50

	FAT GRAMS	PERCENT OF CALORIES FROM FAT
Lemon chiffon / **Pillsbury** No Bake	72	30–40
Vanilla marble / **Pillsbury** No Bake	102	30–40

PIE CRUSTS AND PASTRY SHELLS

	FAT GRAMS	PERCENT OF CALORIES FROM FAT
Pastry sheets, frozen: 1 sheet / **Pepperidge Farm**	45	70–80
Pastry shells: 1 piece / **Stella D'Oro**	8.1	50–60
Patty shells, frozen: 1 shell / **Pepperidge Farm**	19	70–80
Pie crust, mix, prepared: double crust / **Betty Crocker**	128	60–70
Pie crust, mix, prepared: 1 whole crust / **Flako**	84	40–50
Pie crust, mix, prepared: double crust / **Pillsbury**	108	50–60
Pie crust, stick: 1 stick / **Betty Crocker**	72	60–70
Pie shell, dcep, frozen: 1 shell / **Pepperidge Farm**	36	60–70
Pie shell, shallow bottom, frozen: 1 bottom / **Pepperidge Farm**	32	60–70
Pie shell, top, frozen: 1 top / **Pepperidge Farm**	56	60–70
Tart shells, frozen: 1 shell / **Pepperidge Farm**	5	50–60

PIE FILLING

	FAT GRAMS	PERCENT OF CALORIES FROM FAT
Apple: 21 oz can / **Wilderness**	12	10–20
Apple, French: 21 oz can / **Wilderness**	6	0–10
Apricot: 21 oz can / **Wilderness**	6	0–10
Banana cream, mix, prepared for whole 8-in pie / **Jell-O**	18	20–30
Blueberry: 21 oz / **Wilderness**	12	10–20
Cherry: 21 oz can / **Wilderness**	6	0–10

	FAT GRAMS	PERCENT OF CALORIES FROM FAT
Key Lime, mix, prepared: ½ cup / **Royal** Cooked	3	10–20
Lemon: 22 oz can / **Wilderness**	24	20–30
Lemon, mix, prepared: ½ cup / **Royal** Cooked	3	10–20
Mince: 22 oz can / **Wilderness**	30	30–40
Mincemeat: ⅓ cup / **None Such**	2	0–10
Peach: 21 oz can / **Wilderness**	12	10–20
Pumpkin, canned: 1 cup / **Stokely-Van Camp**	0	0–10
Raisin: 22 oz can / **Wilderness**	6	0–10
Strawberry: 21 oz can / **Wilderness**	6	0–10

PIE SNACKS

1 piece

	FAT GRAMS	PERCENT OF CALORIES FROM FAT
Apple pie / **Hostess**	20	40–50
Apple pie / **Tastykake** 4 oz	13	30–40
Apple, French / **Tastykake** 4 oz	14	30–40
Berry / **Hostess**	20	40–50
Blueberry / **Hostess**	20	40–50
Blueberry / **Tastykake** 4 oz	13	30–40
Cherry / **Hostess**	20	40–50
Cherry / **Tastykake** 4 oz	13	30–40
Lemon / **Hostess**	22	40–50
Lemon / **Tastykake** 4 oz	13	30–40
Peach / **Hostess**	20	40–50
Peach / **Tastykake** 4 oz	13	30–40
Pecan: 3 oz / **Frito-Lay**	13.9	30–40

Pizza

1 whole pizza unless noted	FAT GRAMS	PERCENT OF CALORIES FROM FAT
Beef and cheese, frozen / **El Chico** Mexican	60	50–60
Beef and cheese, frozen / **El Chico** Mexican	56	50–60
Canadian bacon, frozen / **Totino's** Party	20	20–30
Cheese		
Frozen: 4 oz / **Buitoni**	8	20–30
Frozen / **Celeste** 7 oz	18	30–40
Frozen / **Celeste** 19 oz	52	30–40
Frozen / **Celeste** Sicilian Style 20 oz	44	20–30
Frozen / **Jeno's** 13 oz	26	20–30
Frozen / **Jeno's** Deluxe 20 oz	57	30–40
Frozen / **La Pizzeria** 20 oz	44	30–40
Frozen, thick crust / **La Pizzeria** 18.5 oz	45	30–40
Frozen: ½ pkg / **Stouffer's**	13	30–40
Frozen / **Totino's** Crisp Party	36	30–40
Frozen / **Totino's** Party	32	30–40
Mix, prepared / **Jeno's**	22	20–30
and mushroom, frozen / **Celeste** 8 oz	8	30–40
and mushroom, frozen / **Celeste** 21 oz	52	30–40
Chili and cheese, frozen / **El Chico** Mexican	58	40–50
Combination		
Frozen / **Celeste** Deluxe 9 oz	32	40–50
Frozen / **Celeste** Deluxe 23½ oz	76	40–50
Frozen / **Jeno's** Deluxe 23 oz	78	40–50
Frozen / **La Pizzeria** 13.5 oz	44	40–50

	FAT GRAMS	PERCENT OF CALORIES FROM FAT
Frozen / **La Pizzeria** 24½ oz	68	40–50
Frozen: ½ pkg / **Stouffer's** Deluxe	18	40–50
Frozen, deep crust / **Totino's** Classic	39	20–30
Frozen / **Totino's** Classic	96	40–50
Hamburger, frozen / **Jeno's**	28	20–30
Hamburger, frozen / **Totino's** Crisp Party	44	40–50
Hamburger, frozen / **Totino's** Party	38	40–50
Open face, frozen: 4 oz / **Buitoni**	5.7	20–30
Pepperoni		
Frozen / **Celeste** 7½ oz	26	40–50
Frozen / **Celeste** 20 oz	76	40–50
Frozen / **Jeno's** 13 oz	30	30–40
Frozen / **La Pizzeria** 21 oz	64	40–50
Frozen: ½ pkg / **Stouffer's**	19	40–50
Frozen, deep crust / **Totino's** Classic	36	10–20
Frozen / **Totino's** Party	36	30–40
Frozen / **Totino's** Crisp Party	46	30–40
Mix, prepared / **Jeno's**	40	30–40
and mushroom, frozen / **Totino's** Classic	72	40–50
Refried bean and cheese, frozen / **El Chico** Mexican	46	40–50
Sausage		
Frozen / **Celeste** 8 oz	30	40–50
Frozen / **Celeste** 22 oz	80	40–50
Frozen / **Jeno's** 13 oz	32	30–40
Frozen / **Jeno's** Deluxe 21 oz	63	30–40
Frozen / **La Pizzeria** 23 oz	80	40–50
Frozen / **La Pizzeria** 13 oz	46	40–50
Frozen, deep crust / **Totino's** Classic	36	10–20
Frozen / **Totino's** Crisp Party	46	40–50
Frozen / **Totino's** Party	36	40–50

	FAT GRAMS	PERCENT OF CALORIES FROM FAT
Mix, prepared / **Jeno's**	44	30–40
and mushroom, frozen / **Celeste** 9 oz	28	40–50
and mushroom, frozen / **Celeste** 21 oz	80	40–50
and mushroom, frozen / **Totino's** Classic	96	50–60
Regular, mix, prepared / **Jeno's**	24	20–30
Pizza Rolls, frozen: 3 oz		
Cheeseburger / **Jeno's**	13	40–50
Pepperoni and cheese / **Jeno's**	14	40–50
Sausage and cheese / **Jeno's**	14	40–50
Shrimp and cheese / **Jeno's**	10	40–50

Popcorn

	FAT GRAMS	PERCENT OF CALORIES FROM FAT
Unpopped: ¼ cup	2.4	10–20
Popped, plain: 1 cup	.3	10–20
Popped, w oil: 1 cup	2	40–50

Pot Pies

	FAT GRAMS	PERCENT OF CALORIES FROM FAT
Frozen: 1 whole pie		
Beef		
Banquet 8 oz	20	40–50
Morton 8 oz	16	40–50
Stouffer's 10 oz	38	60–70
Swanson 8 oz	23	40–50
Swanson Hungry-Man 16 oz	43	50–60
Chicken		
Banquet 8 oz	23.2	40–50
Morton 8 oz	20	40–50
Stouffer's 10 oz	28	50–60
Swanson 8 oz	25	50–60
Swanson Hungry-Man 16 oz	42	40–50
Sirloin Burger / **Swanson** Hungry-Man 16 oz	58	60–70
Tuna / **Banquet** 8 oz	22.9	40–50
Tuna / **Morton** 8 oz	18	40–50
Turkey		
Banquet 8 oz	21.6	40–50
Morton 8 oz	21	40–50
Stouffer's 10 oz	26	50–60
Swanson 8 oz	26	50–60
Swanson Hungry-Man 16 oz	45	50–60

Poultry and Poultry Entrees

FRESH

	FAT GRAMS	PERCENT OF CALORIES FROM FAT
Chicken, broiled: ½ of 1¾ lb broiler	7	20–30
Chicken, fried: parts from 2½ pound fryer		
Back	8.5	50–60
Breast wo ribs: ½ breast	5.1	20–30
Drumstick	3.8	30–40
Neck	7.6	50–60
Rib section: ½ section	2.1	40–50
Thigh	5.9	40–50
Wing	4.5	40–50
Chicken, roasted		
Light meat wo skin: 3½ oz	4.9	20–30
Light meat wo skin, chopped or diced: 1 cup	6.9	20–30
Dark meat wo skin: 3½ oz	6.5	30–40
Dark meat wo skin, chopped or diced: 1 cup	9.1	30–40
Chicken, stewed (hens and cocks)		
Meat and skin: 3½ oz	22.8	60–70
Light meat wo skin: 3½ oz	4.7	20–30
Dark meat wo skin: 3½ oz	9.5	40–50
Chicken livers, raw: 3½ oz	3.7	20–30
Chicken livers, simmered: 3½ oz	4.4	20–30
Duck, domesticated, roasted, meat wo skin: 3½ oz	9.3	40–50
Duck, wild, raw, meat only: 3½ oz	5.2	30–40
Goose, domesticated, roasted meat only: 3½ oz	9.8	30–40

	FAT GRAMS	PERCENT OF CALORIES FROM FAT
meat and skin: 3½ oz	38.1	70–80
Turkey		
Light meat wo skin, roasted: 3½ oz	3.9	10–20
Dark meat wo skin, roasted: 3½ oz	8.3	30–40
Skin only, roasted: 3½ oz	42	80–90
Giblets, simmered: 3½ oz	15.4	50–60

CANNED, FROZEN, AND PROCESSED

	FAT GRAMS	PERCENT OF CALORIES FROM FAT
Chicken a la King, canned: 5¼ oz / **Swanson**	12	50–60
Chicken a la King, frozen: 5 oz / **Banquet** Cookin' Bag	4.7	30–40
Chicken a la King, frozen: 5 oz / **Green Giant** Boil-in-Bag Toaster Toppers	10	50–60
Chicken a la King, frozen: 1 pkg / **Stouffer's** 9½ oz	11	30–40
Chicken, boned white chunk, canned: 2½ oz **Swanson**	5	40–50
Chicken, boned w broth, canned: 2½ oz **Swanson**	6	40–50
Chicken, chopped, pressed: 1 slice / **Eckrich** Slender Sliced	2.8	50–60
Chicken and biscuits, frozen 7 oz / **Green Giant** Oven Baked Entrees	16	70–80
Chicken breast Parmigiana and spinach, frozen: 9 oz / **Weight Watchers**	9	40–50
Chicken, creamed, frozen: 1 pkg / **Stouffer's** 6½ oz	22	60–70
Chicken Creole, frozen / **Weight Watchers** 13 oz	4	10–20
Croquette, chicken w sauce, frozen: 12 oz / **Howard Johnson's**	33.6	50–60

	FAT GRAMS	PERCENT OF CALORIES FROM FAT
Chicken divan, frozen: 1 pkg / **Stouffer's** 8½ oz	22	50–60
Chicken w dumplings, canned: 7½ oz / **Swanson**	12	40–50
Chicken w dumplings, frozen: 32 oz / **Banquet** Buffet Supper	41.8	30–40
Chicken, escalloped, frozen: ½ pkg / **Stouffer's** 11½ oz	15	50–60
Chicken, fried		
Frozen: 6.4 oz / **Morton**	18	30–40
Frozen: 1 entree / **Morton** Country Table 12 oz	25	30–40
Frozen, assorted pieces: 3.2 edible oz / **Swanson**	17	50–60
Frozen, breast portions: 3.2 edible oz / **Swanson**	16	50–60
Frozen, thighs and drumsticks: 3.2 edible oz / **Swanson**	18	60–70
Frozen, wing sections: 3.2 edible oz / **Swanson** Nibbles	20	60–70
Chicken livers w chopped broccoli, frozen: 10½ oz / **Weight Watchers**	5	20–30
Chicken Nibbles w french fries: 1 entree / **Swanson** "TV"	20	40–50
Chicken and noodles, frozen: 32 oz / **Banquet** Buffet Supper	20.9	20–30
Chicken and noodles, frozen: 9 oz / **Green Giant** Boil-In-Bag Entrees	10	30–40
Chicken, smoked, sliced: 1 oz / **Safeway**	3	50–60
Chicken stew, canned: 7½ oz / **Swanson**	7	30–40

	FAT GRAMS	PERCENT OF CALORIES FROM FAT
Chicken, white meat w peas, onion, frozen: 9 oz / **Weight Watchers**	11	30–40
Turkey, boned w broth, canned: 2½ oz / **Swanson**	5	40–50
Turkey slices		
Canned w gravy 6¼ oz / **Morton House**	6	30–40
Frozen entree / **Morton** Country Table 12¼ oz	13	30–40
Frozen entree / **Swanson** Hungry-Man 13¼ oz	13	30–40
Frozen entree: 8¾ oz / **Swanson** "TV"	8	20–30
Frozen w giblet gravy: 5 oz / **Banquet** Cookin' Bag	3.8	30–40
Frozen w giblet gravy: 32 oz / **Banquet** Buffet Supper	17.3	20–30
Frozen w gravy: 5 oz / **Green Giant** Boil-in-Bag Toast Toppers	4	30–40
Turkey Tetrazzini, frozen: ½ pkg / **Stouffer's** 12 oz	14	50–60
Turkey Tetrazzini w mushrooms, red peppers, frozen: 13 oz / **Weight Watchers**	8	10–20
Turkey, roast, frozen, cooked		
Dark meat: 3½ oz / **Swift** Butterball	11	40–50
White meat: 3½ oz / **Swift** Butterball	5	20–30
White and dark meat w skin: 3½ oz / **Swift** Butterball	11	40–50
Roll, boneless white and dark meat: 3½ oz / **Swift** Premium Perfect Slice	2	10–20

	FAT GRAMS	PERCENT OF CALORIES FROM FAT
Roll, white meat: 3½ oz / **Swift** Premium Perfect Slice	1	0–10
Roll, boneless white and dark meat: 3½ oz / **Swift** Park Lane	6	30–40
Roll, white meat, cooked, frozen: 3½ oz / **Swift** Park Lane	6	30–40
Turkey, smoked, chopped: 1 slice / **Eckrich** Slender Sliced	2.8	50–60
Turkey, smoked, sliced: 1 oz / **Safeway**	3	50–60

Pretzels

	FAT GRAMS	PERCENT OF CALORIES FROM FAT
1 oz		
Sticks / **Pepperidge Farm** Thin	1	0–10
Sticks / **Planters**	1	0–10
Twists / **Pepperidge Farm** Tiny	2	10–20
Twists / **Planters**	1	0–10
Twists / **Rold Gold**	1.1	0–10

Pudding

	FAT GRAMS	PERCENT OF CALORIES FROM FAT
½ cup unless noted		
All flavors, mixed prepared / **Estee** Low Calorie	0	0–10
Banana		
Canned, ready to serve: 5 oz can / **Del Monte**	5	20–30
Mix, prepared / **Ann Page**	5	20–30
Mix, prepared / **Jell-O** Instant	5	20–30
Mix, prepared / **Royal** Cooked	4	20–30
Mix, prepared / **Royal** Instant	5	20–30
Butter pecan, mix, prepared / **Jell-O** Instant	5	20–30
Butterscotch		
Canned, ready to serve: 5 oz can / **Del Monte**	5	20–30
Mix, prepared / **Ann Page**	5	20–30
Mix, prepared / **Ann Page** Instant	5	20–30
Mix, prepared with nonfat milk / **D-Zerta**	0	0–10
Mix, prepared / **Jell-O**	5	20–30
Mix, prepared / **Jell-O** Instant	5	20–30
Mix, prepared / **My-T-Fine**	3	10–20
Mix, prepared / **Royal** Cooked	4	20–30
Mix, prepared / **Royal** Instant	5	20–30
Chocolate		
Canned, ready to serve / **Betty Crocker**	5	20–30
Canned, ready to serve: 5 oz can / **Del Monte**	6	20–30
Mix, prepared / **Ann Page**	5	20–30
Mix, prepared / **Ann Page** Instant	5	20–30

	FAT GRAMS	PERCENT OF CALORIES FROM FAT
Mix, prepared with nonfat milk / **D-Zerta**	0	0–10
Mix, prepared / **Jell-O**	5	20–30
Mix, prepared / **Jell-O** Instant	5	20–30
Mix, prepared / **My-T-Fine**	1	0–10
Mix, prepared / **Royal**	4	20–30
Mix, prepared / **Royal** Instant	4	20–30
Almond, mix, prepared / **My-T-Fine**	5	20–30
Fudge, canned, ready to serve / **Betty Crocker**	5	20–30
Fudge, canned, ready to serve: 5 oz can / **Del Monte**	6	20–30
Fudge, mix, prepared / **Jell-O**	5	20–30
Fudge, mix, prepared / **Jell-O** Instant	5	20–30
Fudge, mix, prepared / **My-T-Fine**	3	10–20
Milk, mix, prepared / **Jell-O**	5	20–30
Coconut		
Mix, prepared / **Royal** Instant	4	20–30
Cream, mix, prepared / **Ann Page**	8	30–40
Cream, mix, prepared / **Jell-O**	4	30–40
Cream, mix, prepared / **Jell-O** Instant	7	30–40
Toasted, mix, prepared / **Ann Page**	6	30–40
Coffee, mix, prepared / **Royal** Instant	5	20–30
Custard, mix, prepared / **Royal**	5	20–30
Custard, egg, mix, prepared / **Ann Page**	5	20–30
Custard, egg, mix, prepared / **Jell-O** Americana	6	30–40
Dark 'N Sweet, mix, prepared / **Royal**	4	20–30
Dark 'N Sweet, mix, prepared / **Royal** Instant	4	20–30
Flan, mix, prepared / **Royal**	5	30–40

	FAT GRAMS	PERCENT OF CALORIES FROM FAT
Lemon		
Mix, prepared / **Ann Page**	2	10–20
Mix, prepared / **Ann Page** Instant	5	20–30
Mix, prepared / **Jell-O** Instant	5	20–30
Mix, prepared / **My-T-Fine**	4	20–30
Mix, prepared / **Royal** Instant	5	20–30
Pineapple cream, mix, prepared / **Jell-O** Instant	5	20–30
Pistachio, mix, prepared / **Ann Page** Instant	6	20–30
Pistachio, mix, prepared / **Jell-O** Instant	5	20–30
Pistachio Nut, mix, prepared / **Royal** Instant	4	20–30
Plum Pudding, canned, ready to serve / **R & R**	1.2	0–10
Rice, canned, ready to serve / **Betty Crocker**	4	20–30
Rice, mix, prepared / **Jell-O** Americana	5	20–30
Tapioca		
Canned, ready to serve / **Betty Crocker**	5	20–30
Chocolate, mix, prepared / **Ann Page**	5	20–30
Chocolate, mix, prepared / **Jell-O** Americana	5	20–30
Chocolate, mix, prepared / **Royal**	4	20–30
Vanilla, mix, prepared / **Ann Page**	5	20–30
Vanilla, mix, prepared / **Jell-O** Americana	5	20–30
Vanilla, mix, prepared / **My-T-Fine**	2	10–20
Vanilla, mix, prepared / **Royal**	4	20–30
Vanilla		
Canned, ready to serve / **Betty Crocker**	7	30–40

	FAT GRAMS	PERCENT OF CALORIES FROM FAT
Canned, ready to serve: 5 oz can / **Del Monte**	5	20–30
Mix, prepared / **Ann Page**	5	20–30
Mix, prepared with nonfat milk / **D-Zerta**	0	0–10
Mix, prepared / **Jell-O**	5	20–30
Mix, prepared / **Jell-O Instant**	5	20–30
Mix, prepared / **My-T-Fine**	1	0–10
Mix, prepared / **Royal**	4	20–30
Mix, prepared / **Royal** Instant	5	20–30
French, mix, prepared / **Jell-O**	5	20–30
French, mix, prepared / **Jell-O** Instant	5	20–30

Rice and Rice Dishes

	FAT GRAMS	PERCENT OF CALORIES FROM FAT
Brown, raw: 1 cup	3.5	0–10
Brown, cooked: 1 cup	1.2	0–10
Brown, long grain, parboiled: ⅔ cup cooked / **Uncle Ben's**	1.5	10–20
Brown and wild, seasoned, mix, prepared: ½ cup / **Uncle Ben's**	1.5	10–20
White, raw: 1 cup	.7	0–10
White, cooked: 1 cup	.2	0–10
White: ⅔ cup cooked / **Minute**	0	0–10
White, long grain, parboiled: ⅔ cup cooked / **Uncle Ben's**	.2	0–10
White, precooked: ⅔ cup cooked / **Uncle Ben's** Quick	0	0–10
White and wild, frozen: 1 cup / **Green Giant** Boil-in-Bag	3	10–20
White, long grain and wild, mix, prepared: ½ cup / **Uncle Ben's**	.3	0–10
White, long grain and wild, mix, prepared: ½ cup / **Uncle Ben's** Fast Cooking	.5	0–10
White and wild w bean sprouts, pea pods, and water chestnuts, frozen: 1 cup / **Green Giant** Boil-in-Bag Oriental	5	10–20
White and wild w peas, celery, mushrooms and almonds, frozen: 1 cup / **Green Giant** Boil-in-Bag Medley	12	30–40

	FAT GRAMS	PERCENT OF CALORIES FROM FAT
Beef-flavored, mix, prepared: 1/6 pkg / **Ann Page** Rice 'n Easy	5	20–30
Beef-flavored, mix, prepared: ½ cup / **Minute** Rice Rib Roast	4	20–30
Beef-flavored, mix, prepared: 1/6 pkg / **Rice-A-Roni**	1	0–10
Beef-flavored, mix, prepared: ½ cup / **Uncle Ben's**	.5	0–10
w bell peppers and parsley, frozen: 1 cup / **Green Giant** Boil-in-Bag Verdi	7	20–30
w broccoli, in cheese sauce, frozen: 1 cup / **Green Giant** Boil-in-Bag	8	20–30
Chicken-flavored, mix, prepared: 1/6 pkg / **Ann Page** Rice 'n Easy	6	30–40
Chicken-flavored, mix, prepared: 1/5 pkg / **Rice-A-Roni**	1	0–10
Chicken-flavored, mix, prepared: ½ cup / **Uncle Ben's**	.8	0–10
Curried, mix, prepared: ½ cup / **Uncle Ben's**	.3	0–10
Fried, mix, prepared: ½ cup / **Minute**	5	20–30
w green beans and almonds, frozen: 1 cup / **Green Giant** Boil-in-Bag Continental	8	30–40
and peas w mushrooms, frozen: 2.3 oz / **Birds Eye** Combinations	0	0–10
w peas and mushrooms, frozen: 1 cup / **Green Giant** Boil-in-Bag Medley	5	20–30
Pilaf, mix, prepared: ½ cup / **Uncle Ben's**	.4	0–10

	FAT GRAMS	PERCENT OF CALORIES FROM FAT
Pilaf w mushrooms and onions, frozen:		
1 cup / **Green Giant** Boil-in-Bag	4	10–20
Poultry-flavored, mix, prepared: ½ cup / **Minute** Drumstick	6	30–40
Spanish, mix, prepared: ½ cup / **Minute**	4	20–30
Spanish, mix, prepared: 1/6 pkg / **Rice-A-Roni**	1	0–10
Spanish, mix, prepared: ½ cup / **Uncle Ben's**	.3	0–10

Rolls and Buns

	FAT GRAMS	PERCENT OF CALORIES FROM FAT
1 roll or bun unless noted		
Buns for sandwiches		
Arnold Dutch Egg Buns	3	10–20
Arnold Francisco Sandwich rolls	3	10–20
Arnold Soft Sandwich	2	10–20
w poppy seeds / **Arnold** Soft Sandwich	2	10–20
w sesame seeds / **Arnold** Soft Sandwich	3	20–30
w sesame seeds / **Pepperidge Farm**	3	20–30
Hamburger / **Arnold** 8's	1	10–20
Hamburger / **Pepperidge Farm**	3	20–30
Hamburger / **Wonder**	3	10–20
Hotdog / **Arnold**	1	10–20

	FAT GRAMS	PERCENT OF CALORIES FROM FAT
Hotdog / **Pepperidge Farm**	2	10–20
Hotdog / **Wonder**	3	10–20
Dinner and soft rolls		
Arnold 12's	1.5	20–30
Arnold 24's	1.5	20–30
Arnold Deli-Twist	2	10–20
Arnold Finger 24's	1.5	20–30
Arnold Francisco Variety	1	10–20
Arnold Party Finger 12's	1.5	20–30
Arnold Party Parkerhouse 12's	1.5	20–30
Arnold Party Rounds 12's	1.5	20–30
Arnold Party Tea 20's	.7	20–30
Pepperidge Farm Butter Crescent	7	40–50
Pepperidge Farm Dinner	2	20–30
Pepperidge Farm Finger	1.7	20–30
Pepperidge Farm Finger, sesame	2	30–40
Pepperidge Farm Golden Twist	6	40–50
Pepperidge Farm Old Fashioned	1.3	30–40
Pepperidge Farm Parker House	1.7	20–30
Pepperidge Farm Party	1	20–30
Pepperidge Farm Party Pan	1	20–30
Sara Lee Croissant	6.1	50–60
Sara Lee Parkerhouse Rolls	2.7	30–40
Sara Lee Party Rolls	2	30–40
Sara Lee Poppy Seed Rolls	2	30–40
Sara Lee Sesame Seed Rolls	2	30–40
Wonder Gem Style Dinner	2.5	20–30
Wonder Half and Half Dinner	2.5	20–30
Wonder Home Bake Dinner	2.5	20–30
Wonder Pan	3	20–30
Mix, prepared / **Pillsbury** Hot Roll Mix	2	10–20
Refrigerator / **Ballard** Crescent	4	30–40
Refrigerator / **Pillsbury** Butterflake	3	20–30
Refrigerator / **Pillsbury** Crescent	5	40–50

	FAT GRAMS	PERCENT OF CALORIES FROM FAT
Hard rolls		
Club / **Pepperidge Farm**	1	0–10
Deli / **Pepperidge Farm**	2	0–10
French, four / **Pepperidge Farm**	3	10–20
French, nine / **Pepperidge Farm**	2	10–20
French, large: ½ roll / **Pepperidge Farm**	2	10–20
French, small: ½ roll / **Pepperidge Farm**	1	10–20
French / **Wonder**	2.5	20–30
French sourdough / **Arnold** Francisco	1	0–10
French sourdough / **Arnold** Francisco Brown and Serve	1	0–10
Hearth / **Pepperidge Farm**	1	10–20
Italian: 2 oz / **Pepperidge Farm**	3	10–20
Kaiser and Hoagie rolls: 6 oz / **Wonder**	8	10–20
Sandwich / **Pepperidge Farm**	2	10–20
Sesame Crisp / **Pepperidge Farm**	1.3	10–20
Popovers, mix, prepared: 1 popover / **Flako**	5	20–30

SWEET ROLLS

1 roll unless noted

Apple crunch, frozen / **Sara Lee**	4.7	40–50
Caramel, refrigerated / **Pillsbury** Danish	8	40–50
Caramel, pecan, frozen / **Sara Lee**	8.6	50–60
Caramel sticky buns, frozen / **Sara Lee**	5.7	40–50
Cinnamon, frozen / **Sara Lee**	5.3	40–50
Cinnamon, refrigerated / **Ballard**	3	20–30
Cinnamon w icing, refrigerated / **Hungry Jack Butter Tastin**	6.5	40–50

	FAT GRAMS	PERCENT OF CALORIES FROM FAT
Cinnamon w icing, refrigerated / **Pillsbury**	4	30–40
Cinnamon-raisin, refrigerated / **Pillsbury** Danish	6.5	30–40
Honey Buns / **Hostess**	34	50–60
Honey Buns, frozen / **Morton**	11	40–50
Honey Buns, frozen / **Morton** Mini	5	40–50
Honey Rolls, frozen / **Sara Lee**	5.2	40–50
Orange, refrigerated / **Pillsbury** Danish	4.5	30–40

Salad Dressings

	FAT GRAMS	PERCENT OF CALORIES FROM FAT
Bottled unless noted: 1 tbsp unless noted		
Ann Page Salad Dressing	7	80–90
Mrs. Filbert's Salad Dressing	6	80–90
Nu Made Salad Dressing	7	70–80
Piedmont Salad Dressing	4	50–60
Sultana Salad Dressing	5	80–90
Avocado / **Kraft**	7	80–90
Blue cheese		
Ann Page Low Calorie	1	40–50
Kraft Chunky	6	70–80
Kraft Low Calorie	1	60–70
Kraft Low Calorie Chunky	2	50–60
Kraft Roka	5	70–80
Nu Made	6	70–80
Seven Seas Real	7	80–90
Tillie Lewis / 1 tsp less than 1		0–10
Wish-Bone Chunky	8	80–90
Mix, prepared / **Weight Watchers**	1	80–90
Caesar		
Kraft Golden	7	80–90
Nu Made	8	90–100
Pfeiffer / 1 oz	16	90–100
Pfeiffer Low-Cal / 1 oz	1	40–50
Seven Seas	7	80–90
Wish-Bone	8	80–90
Chef Style / **Ann Page** Low Calorie	1	40–50

	FAT GRAMS	PERCENT OF CALORIES FROM FAT
Chef Style / **Kraft** Low Calorie	1	40–50
Coleslaw Dressing / **Kraft**	6	70–80
Coleslaw Dressing / **Kraft** Low Calorie	2	50–60
Cucumber, creamy / **Kraft**	8	80–90
Cucumber, creamy / **Kraft** Low Calorie	3	80–90
French		
Kraft	6	70–80
Kraft Casino Garlic	6	80–90
Kraft Catalina	5	70–80
Kraft Herb and Garlic	10	90–100
Kraft Low Calorie	2	70–80
Kraft Miracle	6	70–80
Nu Made Low Calorie	1	40–50
Nu Made Savory	6	80–90
Nu Made Zesty	7	90–100
Pfeiffer / 1 oz	10	80–90
Pfeiffer Low-Cal / 1 oz	2	50–60
Seven Seas Creamy	6	80–90
Seven Seas Family Style	6	80–90
Seven Seas Low Calorie	2	50–60
Wish-Bone Deluxe	5	80–90
Wish-Bone Garlic French	6	70–80
Wish-Bone Low Calorie	1	30–40
Wish-Bone Sweet 'n Spicy	6	70–80
Mix, prepared / **Weight Watchers**	0	0–10
French Style / **Ann Page** Low Calorie	2	70–80
French Style / **Kraft** Low Calorie	2	70–80
French Style: 1 tsp / **Tillie Lewis**	less than 1	0–10
Garlic, creamy / **Kraft**	5	80–90
Garlic, creamy / **Wish-Bone**	5	80–90
Green Goddess		
Kraft	9	90–100
Nu Made	6	60–70
Seven Seas	6	80–90

	FAT GRAMS	PERCENT OF CALORIES FROM FAT
Wish-Bone	7	80–90
Green Onion / **Kraft**	8	80–90
Herbs and Spices / **Seven Seas**	6	80–90
Italian		
Ann Page Low Calorie	1	60–70
Kraft	8	80–90
Kraft Golden Blend	7	80–90
Kraft Low Calorie	0	0–10
Nu Made	10	90–100
Nu Made Low Calorie	1	50–60
Pfeiffer Chef / 1 oz	13	90–100
Pfeiffer Low-Cal / 1 oz	1	40–50
Seven Seas	8	90–100
Seven Seas Family Style	7	90–100
Seven Seas Low Calorie	4	90–100
Seven Seas Viva	8	90–100
Tillie Lewis / 1 tsp	0	0–10
Wish-Bone	8	80–90
Wish-Bone Low Calorie	2	80–90
Creamy / **Kraft**	5	80–90
Creamy / **Seven Seas**	7	80–90
Creamy / **Weight Watchers**	5	80–90
Mix, prepared / **Good Seasons**		
Low Calorie	0	0–10
Mix, prepared / **Weight Watchers**	0	0–10
Mix, creamy, prepared /		
Weight Watchers	0	0–10
May Lo Naise / **Tillie Lewis**	3	90–100
Oil and vinegar / **Kraft**	7	80–90
Onion / **Wish-Bone** California	8	80–90
Red Wine: 1 oz / **Pfeiffer** Low-Cal	1	40–50
Russian		
Kraft Low Calorie	1	20–30
Nu Made	5	80–90
Pfeiffer / 1 oz	13	80–90
Pfeiffer Low-Cal / 1 oz	1	20–30

	FAT GRAMS	PERCENT OF CALORIES FROM FAT
Seven Seas Creamy	8	80–90
Tillie Lewis / 1 tsp less than 1		0–10
Weight Watchers	5	80–90
Wish-Bone	3	40–50
Wish-Bone Low Calorie	1	30–40
Creamy / Kraft	6	80–90
w honey / Kraft	5	70–80
Mix, prepared / Weight Watchers	0	0–10
Salad Secret / Kraft	5	70–80
Sour Treat: 1 oz / Friendship	4.4	80–90
Spin Blend / Hellmann's	5	80–90
Thousand Island		
Ann Page Low Calorie	2	70–80
Kraft	6	80–90
Kraft Low Calorie	2	50–60
Nu Made	5	80–90
Nu Made Low Calorie	2	50–60
Pfeiffer / 1 oz	13	80–90
Pfeiffer Low Calorie / 1 oz	1	20–30
Seven Seas	5	80–90
Tillie Lewis / 1 tsp less than 1		0–10
Weight Watchers	5	80–90
Wish-Bone	7	80–90
Wish-Bone Low Calorie	2	70–80
Mix, prepared / Weight Watchers	1	70–80
Vinegar and oil / Nu Made	5	70–80
Vinegar and oil, red wine / Seven Seas Viva	7	80–90
Whipped / Tillie Lewis	3	90–100
Yogonaise / Henri's	6	80–90
Yogowhip / Henri's	5	70–80
Yogurt Blue Cheese / Henri's	2	50–60
Yogurt Creamy Garlic / Henri's	2	50–60
Yogurt Cucumber 'N Onion / Henri's	2	50–60
Yogurt French / Henri's	2	40–50

	FAT GRAMS	PERCENT OF CALORIES FROM FAT
Yogurt Italian / **Henri's**	2	50–60
Yogurt 1000 Island / **Henri's**	2	50–60

Sauces

	FAT GRAMS	PERCENT OF CALORIES FROM FAT
A la King, mix, prepared: ½ cup / **Durkee**	4	50–60
Barbecue, bottled or canned: 1 tbsp		
Chris' and Pitt's	.1	0–10
French's	0	0–10
Open Pit	0	0–10
Hickory smoke flavor / **French's** Smoky	0	0–10
Hot / **French's**	0	0–10
Hot / **Open Pit** Hot 'n Spicy	0	0–10
w onion / **Open Pit**	0	0–10
Cheese, mix, prepared: ½ cup / **Durkee**	10.5	50–60
Cheese, mix, prepared: ¼ cup / **French's**	4	40–50
Hollandaise, mix, prepared: ¾ cup / **Durkee**	14	70–80
Hollandaise, mix, prepared: 3 tbsp / **French's**	4	70–80
Horseradish sauce: 1 tbsp / **Kraft**	5	80–90
Italian, canned: 2 fl oz / **Contadina** Cookbook	1.1	20–30

	FAT GRAMS	PERCENT OF CALORIES FROM FAT
Italian, red, in jar: 5 oz / **Ragu**	2	30–40
Lemon-butter-flavored, mix, prepared: 1 tbsp / **Weight Watchers**	0	0–10
Mushroom steak, canned: 1 oz / **Dawn Fresh**	0	0–10
Pizza, canned: 4 oz / **Buitoni**	5.9	50–60
Pizza, in jar: 5 oz / **Ragu**	6	40–50
Sour cream, mix, prepared: ⅔ cup / **Durkee**	7	20–30
Sour cream, mix, prepared: 2½ tbsp / **French's**	6	90–100
Spaghetti		
Canned: 4 oz / **Ann Page**	2	20–30
Canned: 4 oz / **Buitoni**	4.8	40–50
Canned: ½ cup / **Town House**	4	40–50
In jar: 5 oz / **Ragu** Extra Thick	6	40–50
In jar: 5 oz / **Ragu** Plain	6	50–60
Mix, prepared: 1 env / **Ann Page**	0	0–10
Mix, prepared: ½ cup / **Durkee**	.2	0–10
Mix, prepared: ⅝ cup / **French's** Italian style	4	30–40
Mix, prepared: 4 fl oz / **Spatini**	8	40–50
Clam, canned: 5 oz / **Ragu**	6	40–50
Clam, red, canned: 4 oz / **Buitoni**	4.6	30–40
Clam, white, canned: 4 oz / **Buitoni**	11.6	70–80
Marinara, canned: 4 oz / **Ann Page**	2	20–30
Marinara, canned: 4 oz / **Buitoni**	6.2	60–70
Marinara, in jar: 5 oz / **Ragu**	6	40–50
Meat-flavor, canned: 4 oz / **Ann Page**	3	30–40
Meat-flavor, canned: 4 oz / **Buitoni**	9.1	60–70
Meat flavor, canned: ½ cup / **Town House**	4	40–50
Meat flavor, in jar: 5 oz / **Ragu**	7	50–60
Meat flavor, in jar: 5 oz / **Ragu** Extra Thick	7	40–50

	FAT GRAMS	PERCENT OF CALORIES FROM FAT
w mushrooms, canned: 4 oz / **Ann Page**	2	20–30
w mushrooms, canned: 4 oz / **Buitoni**	5.1	50–60
w mushrooms, in jar: 5 oz / **Ragu**	6	50–60
w mushrooms, in jar: 5 oz / **Ragu** Extra Thick	6	40–50
w mushrooms, canned: ½ cup / **Town House**	4	30–40
w mushrooms, mix, prepared: 1 env / **Ann Page**	0	0–10
w mushrooms, mix, prepared: ⅔ cup / **Durkee**	.2	0–10
w mushrooms, mix, prepared: ⅝ cup / **French's**	4	30–40
Pepperoni flavor, in jar: 5 oz / **Ragu**	7	50–60
Stroganoff		
Mix, prepared: ⅓ cup / **French's**	5	40–50
Mix, prepared, w beef and sour cream: 1 cup / **Durkee**	71.3	70–80
Sweet and sour, canned: 2 fl oz / **Contadina** Cookbook	1.4	10–20
Sweet and sour, canned: 1 cup / **La Choy**	.8	0–10
Sweet and sour, mix, prepared: 1 cup / **Durkee**	5.7	20–30
Sweet and sour, mix, prepared: ½ cup / **French's**	0	0–10
Swiss steak, canned: 2 fl oz / **Contadina** Cookbook	.1	0–10
Teriyaki, mix, prepared: 2 tbsp / **French's**	0	0–10
Tomato, canned		
Contadina / 1 cup	0	0–10
Del Monte / 1 cup	1	10–20
Hunt's / 4 oz	0	0–10

	FAT GRAMS	PERCENT OF CALORIES FROM FAT
Hunt's Prima Salsa Regular / 4 oz	3	20–30
Hunt's Special / 4 oz	0	0–10
Stokely-Van Camp / 1 cup	0	0–10
Town House Spanish style / 8 oz	1	10–20
w bits: 4 oz / **Hunt's**	0	0–10
w cheese: 4 oz / **Hunt's**	2	10–20
w herbs: 4 oz / **Hunt's**	4	40–50
Meat-flavor: 4 oz / **Hunt's** Prima Salsa	3	20–30
w mushrooms: 1 cup / **Del Monte**	1	0–10
w mushrooms: 4 oz / **Hunt's**	0	0–10
w mushrooms: 4 oz / **Hunt's** Prima Salsa	3	20–30
w onion: 1 cup / **Del Monte**	1	0–10
w onions: 4 oz / **Hunt's**	0	0–10
w tidbits: 1 cup / **Del Monte**	1	10–20
White, mix, prepared: ½ cup / **Durkee**	7.5	50–60

Seasoning Mixes

	FAT GRAMS	PERCENT OF CALORIES FROM FAT
Beef stew, mix, prepared: 1 cup / **Durkee**	24	50–60
dry mix: 1 pkg / **Durkee**	.5	0–10
Beef stew: 1 env / **French's**	0	0–10
Burger: ⅓ oz / **Lipton** Make-A-Better-Burger	0	0–10
Chili: 1 env / **Ann Page**	0	0–10

	FAT GRAMS	PERCENT OF CALORIES FROM FAT
Chili: 1 env / **French's** Chilli-O	0	0–10
Chili con carne, prepared: 1 cup / **Durkee**	25	40–50
dry mix: 1 pkg / **Durkee**	1.6	0–10
Chop Suey, prepared: 1 cup / **Durkee**	18.5	50–60
dry mix: 1 pkg / **Durkee**	2.1	0–10
Enchilada, prepared: 1 cup / **Durkee**	.6	0–10
dry mix: 1 pkg / **Durkee**	1.8	0–10
Enchilada: 1 env / **French's**	4	20–30
Fried rice, prepared: 1 cup / **Durkee**	.7	0–10
dry mix: 1 pkg / **Durkee**	1.1	0–10
Ground beef		
Prepared: 1 cup / **Durkee**	48.5	60–70
dry mix: 1 pkg / **Durkee**	.9	0–10
French's Hamburger seasoning: 1 env	0	0–10
w onions: 1 env / **Ann Page**	0	0–10
w onions, prepared: 1 cup / **Durkee**	48	60–70
dry mix: 1 pkg / **Durkee**	0	0–10
w onions: 1 env / **French's**	0	0–10
Hamburger, prepared: 1 cup / **Durkee**	50.5	60–70
dry mix: 1 pkg / **Durkee**	5	40–50
Meatball: 1 env / **French's**	0	0–10
Meatball, Italian, prepared: 1 cup / **Durkee**	48.5	70–80
dry mix: 1 pkg / **Durkee**	.7	20–30
Meatball, Italian w cheese, prepared: 1 cup / **Durkee**	48.5	60–70
dry mix: 1 pkg / **Durkee**	1	10–20
Meatloaf: 1 env / **Contadina**	3.4	0–10
Meatloaf: 1 env / **French's**	0	0–10
Meat marinade, prepared: ½ cup / **Durkee**	.7	10–20
Meat marinade: 1 env / **French's**	0	0–10
Sloppy Joe		
Ann Page / 1 env	0	0–10

	FAT GRAMS	PERCENT OF CALORIES FROM FAT
Durkee / 1 cup prepared	38.8	50–60
dry mix: 1 pkg / **Durkee**	.2	0–10
French's / 1 env	0	0–10
Pizza flavor, prepared: 1 cup / **Durkee**	40.8	60–70
dry mix: 1 pkg / **Durkee**	5	40–50
Spanish rice, prepared: 1 cup / **Durkee**	8.4	20–30
dry mix: 1 pkg / **Durkee**	2.1	10–20
Taco, prepared: 1 cup / **Durkee**	48.6	60–70
dry mix: 1 pkg / **Durkee**	1	10–20
Taco: 1 env / **French's**	0	0–10

Shortening

	FAT GRAMS	PERCENT OF CALORIES FROM FAT
Solid		
Lard: 1 cup	205	100
Lard: 1 tbsp	13	100
Vegetable: 1 tbsp / **Crisco**	12	100
Vegetable: 1 tbsp / **Fluffo**	12	100
Vegetable: 1 tbsp / **Mrs. Tucker's**	13	100
Vegetable: 1 tbsp / **Snowdrift**	12	100

Soft Drinks

No fat

Soups

	FAT GRAMS	PERCENT OF CALORIES FROM FAT
Alphabet vegetable, mix, prepared:		
6 fl oz / **Lipton** Cup-A-Soup	1	20–30
Asparagus, cream of, condensed,		
prepared: 10 oz / **Campbell**	5	40–50
Bean, canned		
Semi-condensed, prepared: 1 can /		
Campbell Soup for One	8	30–40
w bacon, condensed, prepared:		
1 cup / **Ann Page**	5	30–40
w bacon, condensed, prepared:		
10 oz / **Campbell**	6	20–30
w bacon, condensed, prepared:		
1 cup / **Town House**	5.7	30–40
Black, condensed, prepared: 10 oz /		
Campbell	2	10–20
Black, ready to serve: ½ can /		
Crosse & Blackwell	1	0–10
w ham, ready to serve: ½ can		
(9½ oz) / **Campbell** Chunky	10	30–40
w ham, ready to serve: 1 can		
(10¾ oz) / **Campbell** Chunky	11	30–40
w hot dogs, condensed, prepared:		
10 oz / **Campbell**	8	30–40
Beef		
Condensed, prepared: 10 oz /		
Campbell	3	20–30
Ready to serve: ½ can (9½ oz) /		
Campbell Chunky	7	30–40
Ready to serve, individual service		
size: 1 can (10¾ oz) /		
Campbell Chunky	8	30–40

	FAT GRAMS	PERCENT OF CALORIES FROM FAT
Flavor, mix, prepared: 8 oz / **Lipton** Lite-Lunch	7	30–40
Cabbage, condensed, prepared: 8 oz / **Manischewitz**	2.6	30–40
Low sodium, ready to serve, individual service size: 1 can (7¼ oz)/ **Campbell** Chunky	6	30–40
Mushroom, mix, prepared: 8 fl oz / **Lipton**	1	10–20
Noodle, condensed, prepared: 10 oz / **Campbell**	3	20–30
Noodle, condensed, prepared: 1 cup / **Town House**	2.9	30–40
Noodle, mix, prepared: 1 env / **Souptime**	1	20–30
Borscht, condensed, prepared: 8 oz / **Manischewitz**	0	0–10
Borscht, low calorie, condensed, prepared: 8 oz / **Manischewitz**	.1	0–10
Bouillon		
Beef: 1 cube / **Herb-Ox**	0	0–10
Beef: 1 cube / **Maggi**	less than 1	0–10
Beef-flavored: 1 cube / **Wyler's**	less than 1	0–10
Beef-flavored: powder: 1 tsp / **Wyler's** Instant	less than 1	0–10
Chicken: 1 cube / **Herb-Ox**	0	0–10
Chicken: 1 cube / **Maggi**	0	0–10
Chicken-flavored: 1 cube / **Wyler's**	less than 1	0–10
Chicken-flavored, powder: 1 tsp / **Wyler's** Instant	less than 1	0–10
Onion: 1 cube / **Herb-Ox**	0	0–10
Vegetable: 1 cube / **Herb-Ox**	0	0–10

	FAT GRAMS	PERCENT OF CALORIES FROM FAT
Vegetable-flavored, powder: 1 tsp / **Wyler's** Instant	less than 1	0–10
Broth		
Beef: 1 packet / **Herb-Ox**	0	0–10
Beef: 1 tsp / **Herb-Ox** Instant	0	0–10
Beef, canned: 6¾ oz / **Swanson**	1	0–10
Beef, condensed, prepared: 10 oz / **Campbell**	0	0–10
Beef, mix: 1 packet / **Weight Watchers** Broth and Seasoning Mix	0	0–10
Chicken: 1 packet / **Herb-Ox**	0	0–10
Chicken: 1 tsp / **Herb-Ox** Instant	0	0–10
Chicken, canned: 6¾ oz / **Swanson**	2	70–80
Chicken, condensed, prepared: 10 oz / **Campbell**	3	50–60
Chicken, mix, prepared: 6 fl oz / **Lipton** Cup-A-Broth	1	0–10
Chicken, mix: 1 packet / **Weight Watchers**	0	0–10
Onion: 1 packet / **Herb-Ox**	0	0–10
Onion, mix: 1 packet / **Weight Watchers**	0	0–10
Vegetable: 1 packet / **Herb-Ox**	0	0–10
Vegetable: 1 tsp / **Herb-Ox** Instant	0	0–10
Celery, cream of, condensed, prepared: 1 cup / **Ann Page**	3	40–50
Celery, cream of, condensed, prepared: 10 oz / **Campbell**	7	50–60
Celery, cream of, condensed, prepared: 1 cup / **Town House**	6.3	50–60
Cheddar Cheese, condensed, prepared: 10 oz / **Campbell**	12	50–60
Chickarina, canned, ready to serve: 8 fl oz / **Progresso**	5	40–50

	FAT GRAMS	PERCENT OF CALORIES FROM FAT
Chicken		
Canned, ready to serve: ½ can (9½ oz) / **Campbell** Chunky	7	30–40
Canned, ready to serve, individual service size: 1 can (10¾ oz) /**Campbell** Chunky	8	30–40
Flavor, mix, prepared: 8 oz / **Lipton** Lite-Lunch	8	30–40
Alphabet, condensed, prepared: 10 oz / **Campbell**	3	20–30
Barley, condensed, prepared: 8 oz / **Manischewitz**	4.4	40–50
Cream of, condensed, prepared: 1 cup / **Ann Page**	5	40–50
Cream of, condensed, prepared: 10 oz / **Campbell**	9	50–60
Cream of, condensed, prepared: 1 cup / **Town House**	5.3	50–60
Cream of, mix, prepared: 6 fl oz / **Lipton** Cup-A-Soup	3	30–40
Cream of, mix, prepared: 1 env / **Souptime**	6	50–60
w dumplings, condensed, prepared: 10 oz / **Campbell**	7	50–60
Gumbo, condensed, prepared: 10 oz / **Campbell**	2	20–30
Low sodium, ready to serve: 1 can (7½ oz) / **Campbell** Chunky	7	30–40
Noodle, condensed, prepared: 1 cup / **Ann Page**	2	20–30
Noodle, condensed, prepared: 1 cup / **A & P** "O" Style	2	20–30
Noodle, condensed, prepared: 10 oz / **Campbell**	3	20–30
Noodle, condensed, prepared: 10 oz / **Campbell** NoodleO's	3	20–30

	FAT GRAMS	PERCENT OF CALORIES FROM FAT
Noodle, condensed, prepared: 8 oz / **Manischewitz**	2.4	40–50
Noodle, condensed, prepared: 1 cup / **Town House**	2.5	20–30
Noodle, condensed, prepared: 1 cup / **Town House** Star Noodle	2.3	30–40
Noodle, semi-condensed, prepared: 1 can (11⅝ oz) / **Campbell** Soup for One	5	30–40
Noodle, mix, prepared: 6 fl oz / **Lipton** Cup-A-Soup	1	10–20
Noodle, mix, prepared: 8 fl oz / **Lipton** Noodle	2	20–30
Noodle, mix, prepared: 8 fl oz / **Lipton** Ripple Noodle	2	20–30
Noodle, mix, prepared: 1 env / **Souptime**	1	20–30
Rice, canned, ready to serve: ½ can (9½ oz) / **Campbell** Chunky	4	20–30
Rice, condensed, prepared: 1 cup / **Ann Page**	2	20–30
Rice, condensed, prepared: 10 oz / **Campbell**	3	30–40
Rice, condensed, prepared: 8 oz / **Manischewitz**	2.3	40–50
Rice, condensed, prepared: 1 cup / **Town House**	2.7	30–40
Rice, mix, prepared: 8 fl oz / **Lipton**	2	20–30
Rice, mix, prepared: 6 fl oz / **Lipton** Cup-A-Soup	1	10–20
w stars, condensed, prepared: 1 cup / **Ann Page**	2	20–30
w stars, condensed, prepared: 10 oz / **Campbell**	3	30–40

	FAT GRAMS	PERCENT OF CALORIES FROM FAT
Vegetable, canned, ready to serve: ½ can (9½ oz) / **Campbell** Chunky	5	20–30
Vegetable, condensed, prepared: 1 cup / **Ann Page**	3	30–40
Vegetable, condensed, prepared: 10 oz / **Campbell**	4	30–40
Vegetable, condensed, prepared: 8 oz / **Manischewitz**	2.9	40–50
Vegetable, condensed, prepared: 1 cup / **Town House**	3.6	30–40
Vegetable, mix, prepared: 6 fl oz / **Lipton** Cup-A-Soup	1	20–30
Chili beef, condensed, prepared: 10 oz / **Campbell**	8	30–40
Chili beef, condensed, prepared: 1 cup / **Town House**	5.5	20–30
Chili beef, ready to serve: ½ can (9¾ oz) / **Campbell** Chunky	6	20–30
Chili beef, ready to serve: 1 can (11 oz) / **Campbell** Chunky	7	20–30
Chowder		
Clam, prepared: 1 cup / **Howard Johnson's**	7.9	30–40
Clam, ready to serve: 8 fl oz / **Progresso**	1	0–10
Clam, Manhattan, ready to serve: ½ can (9½ oz) / **Campbell** Chunky	4	30–30
Clam, Manhattan, condensed, prepared: 10 oz / **Campbell**	3	20–30
Clam, Manhattan, condensed, prepared: 7 oz / **Snow's**	6	50–60
Clam, Manhattan, ready to serve: ½ can / **Crosse & Blackwell**	1	10–20

	FAT GRAMS	PERCENT OF CALORIES FROM FAT
Clam, New England, condensed, prepared: 10 oz / **Campbell**	3	20–30
made w milk / **Campbell**	8	30–40
Clam, New England, condensed, prepared: 7 oz / **Snow's**	5	30–40
Clam, New England, semi-condensed, prepared: 1 can (11⅝ oz) / **Campbell** Soup for one	4	20–30
Clam, New England, ready to serve: ½ can / **Crosse & Blackwell**	3	50–60
Consommé (beef), condensed, prepared: 10 oz / **Campbell**	1	10–20
Consommé Madrilene, clear, ready to serve: ½ can / **Crosse & Blackwell**	0	0–10
Consommé Madrilene, red, ready to serve: ½ can / **Crosse & Blackwell**	0	0–10
Crab, ready to serve: ½ can / **Crosse & Blackwell**	1	10–20
Escarole, in chicken broth, ready to serve: 1 cup / **Progresso**	2	70–80
Gazpacho, ready to serve: ½ can / **Crosse & Blackwell**	2	50–60
Lentil, ready to serve: 1 cup / **Progresso**	3	10–20
Lentil w ham, ready to serve: ½ can / **Crosse & Blackwell**	2	20–30
Meatball Alphabet, condensed, prepared: 10 oz / **Campbell**	6	30–40
Minestrone		
Condensed, prepared: 1 cup / **Ann Page**	2	20–30
Condensed, prepared: 10 oz / **Campbell**	3	20–30

	FAT GRAMS	PERCENT OF CALORIES FROM FAT
Condensed, prepared: 1 can / **Town House**	6	20–30
Ready to serve: ½ can (9½ oz) / **Campbell** Chunky	4	20–30
Ready to serve: ½ can / **Crosse & Blackwell**	2	10–20
Mushroom		
Condensed, prepared: 10 oz / **Campbell**	5	40–50
Mix, prepared: 1 env / **Souptime**	4	40–50
Barley, condensed, prepared: 8 oz / **Manischewitz**	3.8	40–50
Bisque, ready to serve: ½ can / **Crosse & Blackwell**	5	40–50
Cream of, condensed, prepared: 1 cup / **Ann Page**	7	50–60
Cream of, condensed, prepared: 10 oz / **Campbell**	11	60–70
Cream of, condensed, prepared: 1 cup / **Town House**	8	50–60
Cream of, semi-condensed, prepared: 1 can (11¼ oz) / **Campbell** Soup for One	11	60–70
Cream of, mix, prepared: 6 fl oz / **Lipton** Cup-A-Soup	3	30–40
Cream of, low sodium, ready to serve, individual service size: 1 can (7¼ oz) / **Campbell**	10	60–70
Noodle		
Mix, prepared: 6 fl oz / **Lipton** Cup-A-Soup Giggle	0	0–10
Mix, prepared: 6 fl oz / **Lipton** Cup-A-Soup Ring	1	30–40
Mix, prepared: 8 fl oz / **Lipton** Giggle Noodle	2	20–30

	FAT GRAMS	PERCENT OF CALORIES FROM FAT
Mix, prepared: 8 fl oz / **Lipton** Ring-O-Noodle	1	10–20
w beef flavor, mix, prepared: 6 fl oz / **Lipton** Cup-A-Soup	0	0–10
w chicken, condensed, prepared: 10 oz / **Campbell** Curly	3	20–30
w chicken broth, mix: 1/5 env / **Ann Page**	2	30–40
w chicken broth, mix, prepared: 8 fl oz / **Lipton** Noodle	2	20–30
w ground beef, condensed, prepared: 10 oz / **Campbell**	5	40–50
Onion		
Condensed, prepared: 10 oz / **Campbell**	3	30–40
Mix: 1/5 envelope / **Ann Page**	0	0–10
Mix, prepared: 8 fl oz / **Lipton**	1	20–30
Mix, prepared: 8 fl oz / **Lipton** Beefy	1	20–30
Mix, prepared: 6 fl oz / **Lipton** Cup-A-Soup	1	20–30
Cream of, condensed, prepared: 10 oz / **Campbell**	9	40–50
French, condensed, prepared: 1 can / **Town House**	4	10–20
French, mix, prepared: 1 env / **Souptime**	0	0–10
Mushroom, mix, prepared: 8 fl oz / **Lipton**	1	20–30
Oriental style, mix, prepared: 8 oz / **Lipton** Lite-Lunch	7	20–30
Oyster stew, condensed, prepared: 10 oz / **Campbell**	5	60–70
prepared with milk / **Campbell**	10	50–60
Pea, green		
Condensed, prepared: 10 oz / **Campbell**	4	10–20

	FAT GRAMS	PERCENT OF CALORIES FROM FAT
Mix, prepared: 8 fl oz / **Lipton**	2	10–20
Mix, prepared: 6 fl oz / **Lipton** Cup-A-Soup	1	0–10
Mix, prepared: 1 env / **Souptime**	0	0–10
Low sodium, ready to serve, individual service size: 1 can (7½ oz) / **Campbell**	3	10–20
Pea, split, condensed, prepared: 8 oz / **Manischewitz**	6.2	40–50
Pea, split w ham, condensed, prepared: 1 cup / **Ann Page**	4	10–20
Pea, split w ham, condensed, prepared: 1 cup / **Town House**	2.4	10–20
Pea, split w ham, ready to serve: ½ can (9½ oz) / **Campbell** Chunky	5	10–20
Pea, split w ham and bacon, condensed, prepared: 10 oz / **Campbell**	5	20–30
Pepper Pot, condensed, prepared: 10 oz / **Campbell**	6	40–50
Potato, cream of, condensed, prepared: 10 oz / **Campbell**	3	20–30
prepared w milk / **Campbell**	6	30–40
Potato, cream of, condensed, prepared: 1 can / **Town House**	8	30–40
Schav, condensed, prepared: 8 oz / **Manischewitz**	0	0–10
Scotch Broth, condensed, prepared: 10 oz / **Campbell**	4	30–40
Shrimp, cream of, condensed, prepared: 10 oz / **Campbell**	8	60–70
prepared w milk / **Campbell**	12	50–60
Shrimp, cream, ready to serve: ½ can / **Crosse & Blackwell**	4	30–40

	FAT GRAMS	PERCENT OF CALORIES FROM FAT
Sirloin burger, ready to serve: ½ can (9½ oz) / **Campbell** Chunky	8	30–40
Sirloin burger, ready to serve, individual service size: 1 can (10¾ oz) / **Campbell** Chunky	9	30–40
Steak & potato, ready to serve: ½ can (9½ oz) / **Campbell** Chunky	5	30–40
Stockpot, vegetable, mix, prepared: 8 oz / **Lipton** Lite Lunch	8	30–40
Stockpot, vegetable-beef, condensed, prepared: 10 oz / **Campbell**	5	30–40
Tomato		
Condensed, prepared: 1 cup / **Ann Page**	2	20–30
Condensed, prepared: 10 oz / **Campbell**	2	10–20
prepared w milk / **Campbell**	7	20–30
Condensed, prepared: 1 cup / **Town House**	.7	0–10
Mix, prepared: 6 fl oz / **Lipton** Cup-A-Soup	1	10–20
Mix, prepared: 1 env / **Souptime**	1	10–20
Ready to serve: 8 fl oz / **Progresso**	1	10–20
Beef, condensed, prepared: 10 oz / **Campbell** NoodleO's	5	20–30
Bisque, condensed, prepared: 10 oz / **Campbell**	3	10–20
Low sodium, ready to serve, individual service size: 1 can (7¼ oz) / **Campbell**	4	20–30
Rice, condensed, prepared: 1 cup / **Ann Page**	2	10–20
Rice, condensed, prepared: 10 oz / **Campbell** Old Fashioned	2	10–20

	FAT GRAMS	PERCENT OF CALORIES FROM FAT
Rice, condensed, prepared: 1 can / **Town House**	10	30–40
Royale, semi-condensed, prepared: 1 can / **Campbell** Soup for One	3	10–20
Turkey		
Ready to serve: ½ can (9¼ oz) / **Campbell** Chunky	5	20–30
Noodles, condensed, prepared: 1 cup / **Ann Page**	2	20–30
Noodles, condensed, prepared: 10 oz / **Campbell**	3	30–40
Noodles, condensed, prepared: 1 cup / **Town House**	3.1	30–40
Noodles, low sodium, ready to serve, individual service size: 1 can (7½ oz) / **Campbell**	2	20–30
Vegetable, condensed, prepared: 1 cup / **Ann Page**	2	20–30
Vegetable, condensed, prepared: 10 oz / **Campbell**	4	30–40
Vegetable		
Canned, ready to serve: ½ can (9½ oz) / **Campbell** Chunky	4	20–30
Canned, ready to serve, individual service size: 1 can (10¾ oz) / **Campbell** Chunky	4	20–30
Condensed, prepared: 1 cup / **Ann Page** Vegetarian	2	20–30
Condensed, prepared: 10 oz / **Campbell**	2	10–20
Condensed, prepared: 10 oz / **Campbell** Old Fashioned	4	30–40
Condensed, prepared: 10 oz / **Campbell** Vegetarian	2	10–20
Condensed, prepared: 8 oz / **Manischewitz**	3.5	40–50

	FAT GRAMS	PERCENT OF CALORIES FROM FAT
Condensed, prepared: 1 cup / **Town House** Vegetarian	2	20–30
Semi-condensed, prepared: 1 can / **Campbell** Old World Soup for One	4	20–30
Mix, prepared: 8 fl oz / **Lipton** Country	1	10–20
Mix, prepared: 8 fl oz / **Lipton** Italian	2	10–20
Beef, condensed, prepared: 1 cup / **Ann Page**	3	30–40
Beef, condensed, prepared: 10 oz / **Campbell**	3	20–30
Beef, condensed, prepared: 1 cup / **Town House**	1.5	10–20
Beef, mix, prepared: 8 fl oz / **Lipton**	1	0–10
Beef, mix, prepared: 6 fl oz / **Lipton** Cup-A-Soup	1	10–20
Beef, ready to serve: ½ can (9½ oz) / **Campbell** Chunky	5	20–30
Beef, low sodium, ready to serve: 1 can (7¼ oz) / **Campbell**	3	30–40
Beef w shells, mix, prepared: 8 fl oz / **Lipton**	2	10–20
w beef stock, condensed, prepared: 1 cup / **Ann Page**	2	20–30
w beef stock, condensed, prepared: 1 cup / **Town House**	2.1	20–30
Cream of, mix prepared: 1 env / **Souptime**	4	40–50
Low sodium, ready to serve, individual service size: 1 can (7¼ oz) / **Campbell**	2	10–20
w noodles, condensed, prepared: 10 oz / **Campbell** NoodleO's	3	20–30

	FAT GRAMS	PERCENT OF CALORIES FROM FAT
Spring, mix, prepared: 6 fl oz / **Lipton** Cup-A-Soup	1	10–20
Vichyssoise, ready to serve: ½ can / **Crosse & Blackwell**	4	50–60

Spaghetti and Spaghetti Dishes

	FAT GRAMS	PERCENT OF CALORIES FROM FAT
Plain: 1 cup cooked firm "al dente"	.7	0–10
Plain: 1 cup cooked tender stage	.6	0–10
Spaghetti, in tomato sauce, canned		
Buitoni Twists / ½ can	2	10–20
w cheese: 7⅜ oz / **Franco-American**	2	10–20
w cheese sauce: 7⅜ oz / **Franco-American** "SpaghettiOs"	2	10–20
w frankfurters: 7⅜ oz / **Franco-American** "SpaghettiOs"	10	40–50
w meat sauce: 7¾ oz / **Franco-American**	10	40–50
w meatballs: ½ can / **Buitoni**	9	30–40
w meatballs: ½ can / **Buitoni** Twists	9	30–40
w meatballs: 7¼ oz / **Franco-American**	9	30–40
w little meatballs: 7⅜ oz / **Franco-American** "SpaghettiOs"	9	30–40

	FAT GRAMS	PERCENT OF CALORIES FROM FAT
Spaghetti with sauce, frozen		
Banquet / 3 oz	14.5	40–50
Morton Casserole / 1 pkg	6	20–30
Stouffer's / 1 pkg (14 oz)	12	20–30
w meatballs: 32 oz / **Banquet**		
Buffet Supper	44.5	30–40
w meatballs: 9 oz / **Green Giant**		
Boil-in-Bag Entrees	12	30–40
Spaghetti and sauce, mixes		
Prepared: 1 pouch / **Betty Crocker**		
Mug-O-Lunch	3	10–30
Prepared: 1 cup / **Kraft** Tangy		
Italian Style	6	20–30

Spreads

	FAT GRAMS	PERCENT OF CALORIES FROM FAT
1 oz = about ¼ cup		
Chicken, canned: 1 oz / **Swanson**	5	60–70
Chicken: 1 oz / **Underwood**	4.6	60–70
Chicken salad: 1½ oz / **Carnation**		
Spreadables	7	60–70
Corned beef: 1 oz / **Underwood**	4.3	60–70
Ham, deviled: 1 oz / **Hormel**	6	70–80
Ham, deviled: 1 oz / **Underwood**	9	80–90
Ham salad: 1½ oz / **Carnation**		
Spreadables	5.4	60–70
Liverwurst: oz / **Underwood**	7.8	70–80

	FAT GRAMS	PERCENT OF CALORIES FROM FAT
Peanut butter: 1 tbsp unless noted		
Ann Page Krunchy	8.5	70–80
Ann Page Smooth	8.5	70–80
Ann Page Regular Grind	8.5	70–80
Kitchen King Crunchy	7.5	70–80
Kitchen King Smooth	7.5	70–80
Peter Pan Crunchy	8	70–80
Peter Pan, low sodium	8.5	70–80
Peter Pan, smooth	8	70–80
Planters Creamy	8	70–80
Planters Crunchy	8	70–80
Skippy Creamy, smooth	8.3	70–80
Skippy Old Fashioned Super Chunk	8.2	70–80
Skippy Super Chunk	8.5	70–80
Smucker's Crunchy	7.5	70–80
Smucker's Natural	8	70–80
Smucker's Smooth	7	70–80
Sultana Krunchy	8	70–80
and jelly: 1 oz / **Smucker's** Goober Grape	6	40–50
Roast Beef: 1 oz / **Underwood**	4.3	60–70
Sandwich spread: 1 tbsp unless noted		
Best Foods Spread	6.1	90–100
Hellmann's	6.1	90–100
Kraft	4	70–80
Mrs. Filbert's	4	70–80
Nu Made	5	70–80
Oscar Mayer: 1 oz	5	60–70
Spam, deviled: 1 oz / **Hormel**	7	70–80
Tuna salad: 1½ oz / **Carnation** Spreadables	5.5	60–70
Turkey salad: 1½ oz / **Carnation** Spreadables	5.9	60–70

Sugar and Sweeteners

No fat

Tea

No fat

Toppings

1 tbsp unless noted	FAT GRAMS	PERCENT OF CALORIES FROM FAT
Black cherry: 1 tsp / **No-Cal**	0	0
Black raspberry: 1 tsp / **No-Cal**	0	0
Butterscotch / **Smucker's**	0	0
Caramel / **Smucker's**	0	0
Cherry / **Smucker's**	0	0
Chocolate		
Bosco	.1	0–10
Hershey's	.5	0–10
No-Cal / 1 tsp	0	0–10
Smucker's	1	0–10
Tillie Lewis	0	0–10
Fudge / **Hershey's**	2	30–40
Fudge / **Smucker's**	.5	0–10
Fudge, chocolate mint / **Smucker's**	.5	0–10
Fudge, swiss milk chocolate / **Smucker's**	.5	0–10
Coffee: 1 tsp / **No-Cal**	0	0–10

	FAT GRAMS	PERCENT OF CALORIES FROM FAT
Cola: 1 tsp / **No-Cal**	0	0–10
Peanut butter caramel / **Smucker's**	1	10–20
Pecans in syrup / **Smucker's**	.5	0–10
Pineapple / **Smucker's**	0	0–10
Strawberry: 1 tsp / **No-Cal**	0	0–10
Strawberry / **Smucker's**	0	0–10
Walnuts in syrup / **Smucker's**	.5	0–10
Whipped, non-dairy, frozen / **Cool Whip**	1	60–70
Whipped, mix, prepared / **D-Zerta**	1	90–100
Whipped, mix, prepared / **Dream Whip**	1	90–100

Vegetables

	FAT GRAMS	PERCENT OF CALORIES FROM FAT
Almaranth, raw, leaves: 1 lb	2.3	0–10
Artichokes, cooked, bud or globe: 1 large	.3	0–10
Artichokes, cooked, bud or globe: 1 medium	.2	0–10
Artichokes, cooked, bud or globe: 1 small	.2	0–10
Asparagus, raw, cut: 1 cup	.3	0–10
Asparagus spears, cooked, drained: 1 large	.2	0–10
Asparagus spears, cooked, drained: 1 small	.1	0–10
Bamboo shoots, raw: 1 lb	1.4	0–10
Barley, pearled, light: 1 cup	2	0–10
Barley, pearled, Pot or Scotch: 1 cup	2.2	0–10
Beans		
Great Northern, cooked, drained: 1 cup	1.1	0–10
Lima, immature (green), raw: 1 cup	.8	0–10
Lima, immature (green) cooked, drained: 1 cup	.9	0–10
Lima, mature, cooked, drained: 1 cup	1.1	0–10
Mung, mature, dry, raw: 1 cup	2.7	0–10
Mung, sprouted seeds, raw: 1 cup	.2	0–10

	FAT GRAMS	PERCENT OF CALORIES FROM FAT
Pea, (navy), cooked, drained: 1 cup	1.1	0–10
Pinto, dry, raw: 1 cup	2.3	0–10
Red, kidney, cooked, drained: 1 cup	.9	0–10
Snap, green, cooked, drained: 1 cup	.3	0–10
Snap, yellow or wax, cooked, drained: 1 cup	.3	0–10
White, dry, raw: 1 lb	7.3	0–10
Beets, red, peeled, cooked, drained, whole beets 2-in diam: 2 beets	.1	0–10
Beet greens, cooked, drained: 1 cup	.3	0–10
Broadbeans, immature seeds: 1 lb	1.8	0–10
Broadbeans, mature seeds, dry: 1 lb	7.7	0–10
Broccoli, cooked, drained: 1 large stalk	.8	0–10
Cabbage, raw, shredded: 1 cup	.1	0–10
Carrots, raw 1 carrot (2⅞ oz)	.1	0–10
Cauliflower: 1 head (1.9 lb)	1.7	0–10
Celery: 1 stalk	trace	0–10
Chard, Swiss, cooked, drained, leaves: 1 cup	.4	0–10
Chickpeas or garbanzos, dry, raw: 1 cup	9.6	10–20
Collards, cooked, drained: 1 cup	1.3	0–10
Corn, sweet, white and yellow, cooked, drained: 1 cup	1.7	0–10
Cowpeas, cooked, drained: 1 cup	1.3	0–10
Cucumbers, whole: 1 large	.3	0–10
Dandelion greens, cooked, drained: 1 cup	.6	0–10
Eggplant, cooked, drained, diced: 1 cup	.4	0–10
Kale, cooked, drained: 1 cup	.8	10–20
Lentils, cooked, drained: 1 cup	trace	0–10
Lettuce: 1 head	.3	0–10
Mushrooms: 1 lb	1.4	0–10
Mustard greens, cooked, drained: 1 cup	.6	10–20

	FAT GRAMS	PERCENT OF CALORIES FROM FAT
Okra, cooked, drained: 1 cup	.5	0–10
Onions, raw, chopped: 1 cup	trace	0–10
Parsnips, cooked: 1 large parsnip	.8	0–10
Peas, green, cooked, drained: 1 cup	.6	0–10
Peppers, green: 1 large	.3	0–10
Potatoes, baked in skin: 1 medium potato	.2	0–10
Potato, boiled in skin: 1 medium potato	.1	0–10
Potato, French fried: 10 strips, 2–3½-in long	6.6	40–50
Potatoes, fried from raw: 1 cup	24.1	40–50
Potatoes, mashed w milk and table fat: 1 cup	9	40–50
Radishes, raw, whole: 10 medium	trace	0–10
Rutabagas, cooked, drained: 1 cup	.2	0–10
Soybeans, mature seeds, dry, cooked: 1 cup	10.3	30–40
Soybeans, sprouted seeds, raw: 1 cup	1.5	20–30
Soybean curd (Tofu): 1 piece (2½ x 2¾ x 1 in)	5	50–60
Spinach, raw chopped: 1 cup	.2	0–10
Spinach, cooked, drained: 1 cup	.5	0–10
Squash (Butternut, Acorn, Zucchini, Scallop), cooked: 1 lb	.5	0–10
Squash, Hubbard, baked: 1 lb	1.8	0–10
Sweet potato, baked in skin: 1 potato (5 x 2 in)	.6	0–10
Tomato: 1 large	.2	0–10
Tomato, boiled: 1 cup	.5	0–10
Turnips, cooked, drained: 1 lb	.9	0–10
Turnip greens, cooked, drained: 1 cup	.3	0–10
Water chestnut, Chinese, raw: 1 lb	.7	0–10
Watercress, raw, whole: 1 cup	.1	0–10

CANNED AND FROZEN

	FAT GRAMS	PERCENT OF CALORIES FROM FAT
(⅓ pkg = about ½ cup)		
Artichoke hearts, frozen: 3 oz		
(5 or 6 hearts) / **Birds Eye**	0	0–10
Asparagus, canned: 1 cup		
Cut / **Green Giant**	1	0–10
Cut / **Kounty Kist**	1	0–10
Cut / **Lindy**	1	0–10
Cut / **Stokely-Van Camp**	1	0–10
Spears and tips / **Del Monte**	1	0–10
Spears, tipped / **Del Monte**	1	0–10
Spears / **LeSueur**	1	0–10
Spears / **Town House**	1	0–10
Whole / **Stokely-Van Camp**	1	0–10
White / **Del Monte**	1	0–10
Asparagus, frozen		
Cut: 3.3 oz (about ½ cup) / **Birds Eye**	0	0–10
Cut, in butter sauce: 1 cup / **Green Giant**	6	50–60
Cuts and tips: ½ cup / **Seabrook Farms**	0	0–10
Spears: 3.3 oz (about ½ cup) / **Birds Eye**	0	0–10
Spears: 5 spears / **Seabrook Farms**	0	0–10
Spears, jumbo: 3.3 oz (about ½ cup) / **Birds Eye**	0	0–10
Beans, baked: 1 cup		
Howard Johnson's	10.7	20–30
Pea / **B & M**	8	20–30
Red kidney / **B & M**	8.8	20–30
Yellow eye / **B & M**	10.4	20–30
Beans, baked style: 8 oz unless noted		
w bacon: 7½ oz can / **Hormel Short Orders**	12	30–40

	FAT GRAMS	PERCENT OF CALORIES FROM FAT
In barbecue sauce / **Campbell**	5	10–20
In chili gravy / **Ann Page**	5	10–20
w frankfurters: 7½ oz can / **Hormel Short Orders** Beans 'n Weiners	14	30–40
w frankfurters, in tomato and molasses sauce / **Campbell** Beans and Franks	16	30–40
w ham: 7½ oz can / **Hormel Short Orders**	19	40–50
In molasses and brown sugar sauce / **Campbell** Old Fashioned	5	10–20
w pork and molasses / **Ann Page** Boston Style	5	10–20
w pork and tomato sauce / **Ann Page**	3	10–20
w pork, in tomato sauce / **Campbell**	4	10–20
In tomato sauce / **Ann Page** Vegetarian	1	0–10
In tomato sauce / **Morton** House	4	10–20
Beans, black turtle, canned: 1 cup / **Progresso**	1	0–10
Beans, fava, canned: 1 cup / **Progresso**	1	0–10
Beans, green, canned: 1 cup		
Cut / **Del Monte**	0	0–10
Cut / **Green Giant**	0	0–10
Cut / **Kounty Kist**	0	0–10
Cut / **Libby's**	0	0–10
Cut / **Lindy**	0	0–10
Cut / **Stokely-Van Camp**	0	0–10
French, cut / **Del Monte**	0	0–10
French / **Green Giant**	0	0–10
French / **Kounty Kist**	0	0–10
French / **Libby's** Blue Lake	0	0–10
French / **Lindy**	0	0–10

	FAT GRAMS	PERCENT OF CALORIES FROM FAT
Italian / **Del Monte**	0	0–10
Seasoned / **Del Monte**	0	0–10
Sliced / **Stokely-Van Camp**	0	0–10
Whole / **Del Monte**	0	0–10
Whole, tiny / **Del Monte**	0	0–10
Whole / **Green Giant**	0	0–10
Whole / **Kounty Kist**	0	0–10
Whole / **Libby's**	0	0–10
Whole / **Lindy**	0	0–10
Whole / **Stokely-Van Camp**	0	0–10
Beans, green, frozen		
Cut: 3 oz (about ½ cup) / **Birds Eye**	0	0–10
Cut: 1 cup / **Kounty Kist** Poly Bag	0	0–10
Cut: ½ cup / **Seabrook Farms**	0	0–10
Cut, in butter sauce: 1 cup / **Green Giant**	4	50–60
French: 3 oz (about ½ cup) / **Birds Eye**	0	0–10
French: ½ cup / **Seabrook Farms**	0	0–10
French, in butter sauce: 1 cup / **Green Giant**	4	50–60
French w sliced mushrooms: 3 oz (about ½ cup) / **Birds Eye**	0	0–10
French w toasted almonds: 3 oz (about ½ cup) / **Birds Eye**	2	30–40
Italian: 3 oz / **Birds Eye**	0	0–10
w onions and bacon bits: 1 cup / **Green Giant**	4	30–40
and pearl onions: 3 oz (about ½ cup) / **Birds Eye**	0	0–10
and spaetzle w sauce: 3.3 oz (about ½ cup) / **Birds Eye**	1	10–20
Whole: 3 oz (about ½ cup) / **Birds Eye**	0	0–10
Beans, kidney, red: 8 oz / **Ann Page**	1	0–10
Beans, kidney, red: 1 cup / **Progresso**	1	0–10

	FAT GRAMS	PERCENT OF CALORIES FROM FAT
Beans, kidney, white, canned: 1 cup / **Progresso** Cannellini	1	0–10
Beans, lima		
Baby, canned: 8 oz / **Sultana**	1	0–10
Baby, frozen: 3.3 oz (about ½ cup) / **Birds Eye**	1	0–10
Baby, frozen: 1 cup / **Green Giant** Poly Bag	1	0–10
Baby, frozen: 1 cup / **Kounty Kist** Poly Bag	1	0–10
Baby, frozen: ½ cup / **Seabrook Farms**	1	0–10
Baby, in butter sauce, frozen: 1 cup / **Green Giant**	6	20–30
Canned: 1 cup / **Del Monte**	1	0–10
Canned: 1 cup / **Libby's**	1	0–10
Canned: 1 cup / **Stokely-Van Camp**	1	0–10
Canned, seasoned: 1 cup / **Del Monte**	1	0–10
Fordhook, frozen: 3.3 oz (about ½ cup) / **Birds Eye**	0	0–10
Fordhook, frozen: ½ cup / **Seabrook Farms**	0	0–10
Tiny, frozen: 3.3 oz (about ½ cup) / **Birds Eye**	1	0–10
Beans, pinto, canned: 1 cup / **Progresso**	1	0–10
Beans, red, canned: 8 oz / **Ann Page**	1	0–10
Beans, Roman, canned: 1 cup / **Progresso**	1	0–10
Beans, salad, canned: 1 cup / **Green Giant** 3-Bean	1	0–10
Beans, Shellie, canned: 1 cup / **Stokely-Van Camp**	0	0–10
Beans, wax or yellow: 1 cup unless noted		
Cut, canned / **Del Monte**	0	0–10

	FAT GRAMS	PERCENT OF CALORIES FROM FAT
French cut, canned / **Del Monte**	0	0–10
Cut, canned / **Libby's**	0	0–10
Cut, canned / **Stokely-Van Camp**	0	0–10
Cut, frozen: 3 oz (about ½ cup) / **Birds Eye**	0	0–10
Cut, frozen: ½ cup / **Seabrook Farms**	0	0–10
Sliced, canned / **Stokely-Van Camp**	0	0–10
Beets: 1 cup unless noted		
Cut, canned / **Del Monte**	0	0–10
Cut, canned / **Libby's**	0	0–10
Cut, canned / **Stokely-Van Camp**	0	0–10
Diced, canned / **Libby's**	0	0–10
Diced, canned / **Stokely-Van Camp**	0	0–10
Harvard, canned / **Stokely-Van Camp**	1	0–10
Harvard, diced, canned / **Libby's**	0	0–10
Pickled, crinkle cut, canned / **Del Monte**	0	0–10
Pickled, sliced, canned / **Libby's**	0	0–10
Pickled, sliced, canned / **Stokely-Van Camp**	0	0–10
Pickled, sliced, canned / **Town House**	0	0–10
Pickled, whole, canned / **Libby's**	0	0–10
Pickled, whole, canned / **Stokely-Van Camp**	0	0–10
Shoestring, canned / **Libby's**	0	0–10
Sliced, canned / **Del Monte**	0	0–10
Sliced, canned / **Libby's**	0	0–10
Sliced, canned: ½ cup / **S and W Nutradiet**	0	0–10
Sliced, canned / **Stokely-Van Camp**	0	0–10
Whole, canned / **Del Monte**	0	0–10
Whole, canned / **Libby's**	0	0–10
Whole, canned / **Stokely-Van Camp**	0	0–10

	FAT GRAMS	PERCENT OF CALORIES FROM FAT
Broccoli, frozen		
Au gratin: ½ pkg / **Stouffer's**	12	60–70
w cauliflower and carrots, in cheese		
sauce: 1 cup / **Green Giant**	6	30–40
w cheese sauce: 3.3 oz (about ½		
cup) / **Birds Eye**	8	60–70
w cheese sauce: 1 cup / **Green Giant**	6	40–50
w cheese sauce: 1 cup /		
Green Giant Bake n' Serve	18	60–70
Chopped: 3.3 oz (about ½ cup) /		
Birds Eye	0	0–10
Chopped: ½ cup / **Seabrook Farms**	0	0–10
Cut: 1 cup / **Green Giant** Poly Bag	0	0–10
Cut: 1 cup / **Kounty Kist** Poly Bag	0	0–10
Spears: 3.3 oz / **Birds Eye**	0	0–10
Spears: ⅓ pkg / **Seabrook Farms**	0	0–10
Spears, baby: 3.3 oz / **Birds Eye**	0	0–10
Spears, in butter sauce: 1 cup /		
Green Giant	5	40–50
Brussels sprouts, frozen: 1 cup unless noted		
Birds Eye / 3.3 oz	0	0–10
Green Giant Poly Bag	0	0–10
Kounty Kist Poly Bag	0	0–10
Seabrook Farms / ½ cup	0	0–10
Baby: 3.3 oz / **Birds Eye**	0	0–10
In butter sauce / **Green Giant**	5	40–50
Halves, in cheese sauce /		
Green Giant	7	30–40
Butterbeans, canned: 8 oz / **Sultana**	1	0–10
Butterbeans, baby, frozen: 3.3 oz /		
Birds Eye	0	0–10
Butterbeans, baby frozen: ½ cup /		
Seabrook Farms	1	0–10
Butterbeans, speckled, frozen: 1 cup /		
Green Giant Boil-in-Bag		
Southern Recipe	11	30–40

	FAT GRAMS	PERCENT OF CALORIES FROM FAT
Butterbeans, speckled, frozen:		
½ cup / **Seabrook Farms**	0	0–10
Carrots: 1 cup unless noted		
Cut, canned: ½ cup / **S and W**		
Nutradiet	0	0–10
Diced, canned / **Del Monte**	0	0–10
Diced, canned / **Libby's**	0	0–10
Diced, canned / **Stokely-Van Camp**	0	0–10
Sliced, canned / **Del Monte**	0	0–10
Sliced, canned / **Libby's**	0	0–10
Sliced, canned / **Stokely-Van Camp**	0	0–10
w brown sugar glaze, frozen:		
3.3 oz / **Birds Eye**	2	20–30
In butter sauce, frozen /		
Green Giant Nuggets	5	40–50
Cauliflower, frozen: 1 cup unless noted		
Birds Eye / 3.3 oz	0	0–10
Green Giant Poly Bag	0	0–10
Kounty Kist Poly Bag	0	0–10
Seabrook Farms / ½ cup	0	0–10
w cheese sauce: 3.3 oz / **Birds Eye**	7	50–60
In cheese sauce / **Green Giant**	6	40–50
In cheese sauce / **Green Giant**		
Bake n' Serve	15	60–70
Chick peas, canned: 1 cup / **Progresso**	3	10–20
Collard greens, frozen: ½ cup /		
Seabrook Farms	0	0–10
Collard greens, frozen, chopped:		
3.3 oz / **Birds Eye**	0	0–10
Corn, golden, canned: 1 cup		
Cream style / **Del Monte**	1	0–10
Cream Style / **Green Giant**	2	0–10
Cream style / **Kounty Kist**	2	0–10
Cream style / **Lindy**	2	0–10
Cream style / **Stokely-Van Camp**	1	0–10

	FAT GRAMS	PERCENT OF CALORIES FROM FAT
Liquid pack / **Del Monte** Family style	1	0–10
Liquid pack / **Green Giant**	1	0–10
Liquid pack / **Kounty Kist**	1	0–10
Liquid pack / **Le Sueur**	1	0–10
Liquid pack / **Lindy**	1	0–10
Liquid pack / **Stokely-Van Camp**	1	0–10
Vacuum pack / **Del Monte**	1	0–10
Vacuum pack / **Green Giant** Niblets	1	0–10
Vacuum pack / **Kounty Kist**	1	0–10
Vacuum pack / **Stokely-Van Camp**	1	0–10
Vacuum pack / **Lindy**	1	0–10
w peppers / **Del Monte** Corn 'n Peppers	1	0–10
w peppers / **Green Giant** Mexicorn	1	0–10
Corn, golden, frozen		
In butter sauce: 1 cup / **Green Giant** Niblets	6	20–30
On cob: 1 ear / **Birds Eye**	1	0–10
On cob: 1 ear / **Birds Eye** Little Ears	1	0–10
On cob: 1 ear / **Green Giant**	1	0–10
On cob: 1 ear / **Green Giant** Nibbler	1	0–10
On cob: 1 ear / **Seabrook Farms**	1	0–10
Cream style: 1 cup / **Green Giant**	1	0–10
w peppers in butter sauce: 1 cup / **Green Giant** Mexican	6	20–30
Souffle: ⅓ pkg / **Stouffer's**	7	40–50
Whole kernel: 3.3 oz / **Birds Eye**	0	0–10
Whole kernel: 1 cup / **Green Giant** Poly Bag	1	0–10
Whole kernel: 1 cup / **Kounty Kist** Poly Bag	1	0–10
Whole kernel: 3 oz / **Ore-Ida**	1	0–10

	FAT GRAMS	PERCENT OF CALORIES FROM FAT
Whole kernel: ½ cup / **Seabrook Farms**	1	0–10
Corn, white: 1 cup		
Cream style, canned / **Del Monte**	1	0–10
Cream style, canned / **Stokely-Van Camp**	1	0–10
Whole kernel, canned / **Del Monte**	1	0–10
Whole kernel, canned, vacuum pack / **Green Giant**	1	0–10
Whole kernel, frozen / **Green Giant** Poly Bag	1	0–10
Whole kernel, frozen / **Kounty Kist** Poly Bag	1	0–10
Whole kernel, in butter sauce, frozen / **Green Giant**	6	20–30
Eggplant Parmesan, frozen: 5½ oz / **Mrs. Paul's**	16	50–60
Eggplant sticks, fried, frozen: 3½ oz / **Mrs. Paul's**	15	50–60
Eggplant slices, fried, frozen: 3 oz / **Mrs. Paul's**	15	50–60
Green peppers, stuffed, frozen: 1 pkg / **Stouffer's**	11	40–50
Green peppers, stuffed, frozen: 13 oz / **Weight Watchers**	9	20–30
Kale, chopped, frozen: 3.3 oz (about ½ cup) / **Birds Eye**	0	0–10
Kale, chopped, frozen: ½ cup / **Seabrook Farms**	0	0–10
Mixed, canned: 1 cup / **Del Monte**	1	0–10
Mixed, canned: 1 cup / **Stokely-Van Camp**	0	0–10
Mixed, canned: 1 cup / **Town House**	1	0–10
Mixed, frozen: 3.3 oz unless noted **Birds Eye**	0	0–10

	FAT GRAMS	PERCENT OF CALORIES FROM FAT
Green Giant Poly Bag / 1 cup	1	0–10
Kounty Kist Poly Bag / 1 cup	1	0–10
California blend: 1 cup / **Kounty Kist** Poly Bag	0	0–10
Cantonese style / **Birds Eye** Stir Fry	0	0–10
Chinese: 1 cup / **Green Giant** Boil-in-Bag Oriental Combination	4	20–30
Chinese: 1 pkg / **La Choy**	.9	0–10
Chinese w sauce / **Birds Eye** International	0	0–10
Chinese w seasonings / **Birds Eye** Stir-Fry	0	0–10
Danish style w sauce / **Birds Eye** International	0	0–10
Hawaiian style / **Birds Eye** International	0	0–10
Hawaiian style: 1 cup / **Green Giant** Boil-in-Bag Oriental Combination	7	30–40
Italian style w sauce / **Birds Eye** International	1	0–10
Japanese: 1 pkg / **La Choy**	0	0–10
Japanese style: 1 cup / **Green Giant** Boil-in-Bag Oriental Combination	3	20–30
Japanese style w sauce / **Birds Eye** International	0	0–10
Japanese style w seasonings / **Birds Eye** Stir-Fry	0	0–10
Jubilee / **Birds Eye Combinations**	5	30–40
Mandarin style w seasonings / **Birds Eye** Stir-Fry	0	0–10

	FAT GRAMS	PERCENT OF CALORIES FROM FAT
New England style / **Birds Eye** Americana Recipe	1	0–10
New Orleans Creole style / **Birds Eye** Americana Recipe	0	0–10
Parisian style w sauce / **Birds Eye** International	0	0–10
Pennsylvania Dutch style / **Birds Eye** Americana Recipe	1	0–10
San Francisco style / **Birds Eye** Americana Recipe	1	0–10
Wisconsin country style / **Birds Eye** Americana Recipe	1	0–10
In butter sauce: 1 cup / **Green Giant**	5	30–40
In onion sauce: 2.6 oz / **Birds Eye**	5	40–50
Mushrooms		
Canned: 4 oz can / **Dole**	0	0–10
Pieces and stems, canned: 1 oz / **Green Giant**	0	0–10
Sliced, canned: 1 oz / **Green Giant**	0	0–10
Whole, canned: 1 oz / **Green Giant**	0	0–10
In butter sauce, frozen: 2 oz / **Green Giant**	2	50–60
Mustard greens, chopped, frozen: 3.3 oz / **Birds Eye**	0	0–10
Mustard greens, chopped: ½ cup / **Seabrook Farms**	0	0–10
Okra, cut, frozen: 3.3 oz / **Birds Eye**	0	0–10
Okra, cut, frozen: ½ cup / **Seabrook Farms**	0	0–10
Okra Gumbo, frozen: 1 cup / **Green Giant** Boil-in-Bag Southern Recipe	18	70–80
Okra, whole, frozen: 3.3 oz / **Birds Eye**	0	0–10
Okra, whole, frozen: ½ cup / **Seabrook Farms**	0	0–10

	FAT GRAMS	PERCENT OF CALORIES FROM FAT
Onions, boiled, canned: 4 oz / **O & C**	0	0–10
Onions, in cream sauce, canned:		
1 oz / **O & C**	.3	0-10
Onions, frozen		
Chopped: 1 oz / **Birds Eye**	0	0–10
Chopped: 1 oz / **Ore-Ida**	0	0–10
Small, whole: 3.3 oz / **Birds Eye**	0	0–10
In cheese flavor sauce: 1 cup /		
Green Giant	8	50–60
In cream sauce: 3 oz / **Birds Eye**	6	50–60
Onion rings, fried, frozen: 2½ oz /		
Mrs. Paul's	7	40–50
Onion rings, fried, canned: 1 oz /		
O & C	15	70–80
Onion rings, fried, frozen:		
2 oz / **Ore-Ida** Onion Ringers	11	40–50
Peas, black-eye		
Canned: 1 cup / **Progresso**	1	0–10
Canned w pork: 8 oz / **Sultana**	4	10–20
Frozen: 3.3 oz / **Birds Eye**	0	0–10
Frozen: 1 cup / **Green Giant**		
Boil-in-Bag Southern Recipe	12	30–40
Frozen: ½ cup / **Seabrook Farms**	0	0–10
Peas, green, canned: 1 cup		
April Showers	1	0–10
Early / **Del Monte**	1	0–10
Early / **Kounty Kist**	1	0–10
Early, small / **Le Sueur**	1	0–10
Early / **Lindy**	1	0–10
Early / **Minnesota Valley**	1	0–10
Early / **Stokeley-Van Camp**	1	0–10
Seasoned / **Del Monte**	1	0–10
Sweet, tiny / **Del Monte**	1	0–10
Sweet / **Green Giant**	1	0–10
Sweet, small / **Green Giant**		
Sweetlets	1	0–10

	FAT GRAMS	PERCENT OF CALORIES FROM FAT
Sweet / **Kounty Kist**	1	0–10
Sweet / **Le Sueur**	1	0–10
Sweet / **Lindy**	1	0–10
Sweet / **Stokely-Van Camp**	1	0–10
Sweet w onions / **Green Giant**	1	0–10
Early w onions / **Green Giant**	1	0–10
and carrots / **Del Monte**	0	0–10
and carrots / **Stokely-Van Camp**	1	0–10
Peas, green, frozen		
Early: 3.3 oz / **Birds Eye**	0	0–10
Early: 1 cup / **Green Giant** Poly Bag	1	0–10
Early: 1 cup / **Kounty Kist** Poly Bag	1	0–10
Early, in butter sauce: 1 cup / **Le Sueur**	5	20–30
Sweet: 1 cup / **Green Giant** Poly Bag	1	0–10
Sweet: ½ cup / **Seabrook Farms**	0	0–10
Sweet, in butter sauce: 1 cup / **Green Giant**	6	30–40
Tiny: 3.3 oz / **Birds Eye**	0	0–10
and carrots: 3.3 oz / **Birds Eye**	0	0–10
and carrots: 1 cup / **Kounty Kist** Poly Bag	2	10–20
and cauliflower w cream sauce: 3.3 oz / **Birds Eye** Combinations	5	40–50
w cream sauce: 2.6 oz / **Birds Eye** Combinations	7	50–60
Creamed w bread crumb topping: 1 cup / **Green Giant** Bake n' Serve	15	20–30
w onions and carrots in butter sauce: 1 cup / **Le Sueur**	6	30–40

	FAT GRAMS	PERCENT OF CALORIES FROM FAT
w pea pods and water chestnuts in sauce: 1 cup / **Le Sueur**	8	30–40
and pearl onions: 3.3 oz / **Birds Eye** Combinations	0	0–10
and potatoes w cream sauce: 2.6 oz / **Birds Eye** Combinations	7	40–50
w sliced mushrooms: 3.3 oz / **Birds Eye** Combinations	0	0–10
Potatoes au gratin w bacon, canned: 7½ oz can / **Hormel Short Orders**	13	40–50
Potatoes, new, canned: 1 cup / **Del Monte**	0	0–10
Potatoes, scalloped w ham, canned: 7½ oz can / **Hormel Short Orders**	16	50–60
Potatoes, whole, canned: 1 cup / **Stokely-Van Camp**	1	0–10
Potatoes, frozen		
Au gratin, 1 cup / **Green Giant** Bake n' Serve	25	50–60
Au gratin: ⅓ pkg /**Stouffer's**	8	50–60
Diced, in sour cream sauce: 1 cup / **Green Giant** Boil-in-Bag	11	30–40
French-fried: 2.8 oz / **Birds Eye** Cottage Fries	5	30–40
French fried: 3 oz / **Birds Eye** Crinkle Cuts	4	30–40
French fried: 3 oz / **Birds Eye** Deep Gold Crinkle Cuts	3	20–30
French fried: 3 oz / **Birds Eye** French Fries	4	30–40
French fried: 3.3 oz / **Birds Eye** Shoestrings	6	30–40

	FAT GRAMS	PERCENT OF CALORIES FROM FAT
French fried: 3 oz / **Birds Eye** Steak Fries	3	20–30
French fried: 3 oz / **Ore-Ida** Cottage Fries	5	30–40
French fried: 3 oz / **Ore-Ida** Country Style Dinner Fries	5	30–40
French fried: 3 oz / **Ore-Ida** Crispers	15	50–60
French fried: 3 oz / **Ore-Ida** Golden Crinkles	5	30–40
French fried: 3 oz / **Ore-Ida** Golden Fries	5	30–40
French fried: 3 oz / **Ore-Ida** Pixie Crinkles	7	30–40
French fried: 3 oz / **Ore-Ida** Self Sizzling Crinkles	7	30–40
French fried: 3 oz / **Ore-Ida** Self Sizzling Fries	9	30–40
French fried: 3 oz / **Ore-Ida** Self Sizzling Shoestrings	11	40–50
French fried: 3oz / **Ore-Ida** Shoestrings	7	30–40
Fried: 3 oz / **Birds Eye** Deep Gold	6	30–40
Fried: 2.5 oz / **Birds Eye** Tasti Fries	7	40–50
Fried: 2.5 oz / **Birds Eye** Tasti Puffs	12	50–60
Fried: 3.2 oz / **Birds Eye** Tiny Taters	12	50–60
Hash browns: 4 oz / **Birds Eye**	0	0–10
Hash browns: 4 oz /**Birds Eye** O'Brien	0	0–10
Hash browns: 3 oz / **Ore-Ida** Southern Style	0	0–10
Hash browns w butter sauce: 3 oz / **Ore-Ida** Southern Style	6	40–50

	FAT GRAMS	PERCENT OF CALORIES FROM FAT
Hash browns w butter sauce and onions: 3 oz / **Ore-Ida** Southern Style	8	50–60
Hash browns, shredded: 3 oz / **Birds Eye**	0	0–10
Hash browns, shredded: 3 oz / **Ore-Ida**	0	0–10
O'Brien: 3 oz / **Ore-Ida**	0	0–10
Scalloped: ⅓ pkg / **Stouffer's**	7	40–50
Shoestring in butter sauce: 1 cup / **Green Giant** Boil-in-Bag	17	40–50
Slices in butter sauce: 1 cup / **Green Giant** Boil-in-Bag	10	40–50
Stuffed w cheese-flavored topping: 5 oz / **Green Giant** Oven Bake	12	40–50
Stuffed w sour cream and chives: 5 oz / **Green Giant** Oven Bake	10	30–40
and sweet peas in bacon cream sauce: 1 cup / **Green Giant** Boil-in-Bag	10	30–40
Tater Tots: 3 oz / **Ore-Ida**	7	30–40
Tater Tots w bacon flavor: 3 oz / **Ore-Ida**	7	30–40
Tater Tots w onions: 3 oz / **Ore-Ida**	7	30–40
Vermicelli: 1 cup / **Green Giant** Bake n' Serve	20	40–50
Whole, boiled: ½ cup / **Seabrook Farms**	0	0–10
Whole peeled: 3.2 oz / **Birds Eye**	0	0–10
Whole, small, peeled: 3 oz / **Ore-Ida**	0	0–10
Potatoes, mix, prepared: ½ cup unless noted		
Au gratin / **Betty Crocker**	6	30–40
Au gratin / **French's** Big Tate	6	20–30
Creamed / **Betty Crocker**	7	30–40

	FAT GRAMS	PERCENT OF CALORIES FROM FAT
Hash brown / **French's** Big Tate	8	40–50
Hash brown w onions /		
Betty Crocker	6	30–40
Julienne / **Betty Crocker**	6	30–40
Mashed / **Betty Crocker**		
Potato Buds	6	40–50
Mashed / **French's**	6	40–50
Mashed / **French's** Big Tate	7	40–50
Mashed / **Hungry Jack** (4 serving		
container)	10	50–60
(12, 24, 40 serving container)	7	40–50
Mashed / **Magic Valley**	4	30–40
Pancakes: three 3-in cakes /		
French's Big Tate	5	30–40
Scalloped / **Betty Crocker**	6	30–40
Scalloped / **French's** Big Tate	6	20–30
w sour cream and chives /		
Betty Crocker Sour Cream		
'n Chive	6	30–40
Potatoes, sweet, frozen		
Candied: 4 oz / **Mrs. Paul's**	0	0–10
Candied w apples: 4 oz /		
Mrs. Paul's	1	0–10
Candied, orange: 4 oz /		
Mrs. Paul's	0	0–10
Glazed: 1 cup / **Green Giant**		
Boil-in-Bag Southern Recipe	8	20–30
Pumpkin, canned: 1 cup / **Del Monte**	1	0–10
Pumpkin, canned: 1 cup /		
Stokely-Van Camp	1	0–10
Sauerkraut, canned: 1 cup		
Del Monte	0	0–10
Libby's	0	0–10
Chopped / **Stokely-Van Camp**	0	0–10
Shredded / **Stokely-Van Camp**	0	0–10
Soup Greens, in jar: 1 jar / **Durkee**	3	10–20

	FAT GRAMS	PERCENT OF CALORIES FROM FAT
Spinach, canned: 1 cup / **Del Monte**	1	0–10
Spinach, frozen		
In butter sauce: 1 cup / **Green Giant**	5	40–50
Chopped: 3.3 oz / **Birds Eye**	0	0–10
Chopped: ½ cup / **Seabrook Farms**	0	0–10
Creamed: 3 oz / **Birds Eye** Combinations	4	50–60
Creamed: 1 cup / **Green Giant**	9	40–50
Leaf: 3.3 oz / **Birds Eye**	0	0–10
Leaf: ½ cup / **Seabrook Farms**	0	0–10
Souffle: 1 cup / **Green Giant** Bake n' serve	17	50–60
Souffle: ⅓ pkg / **Stouffer's**	7	40–50
Squash, cooked, frozen: 4 oz / **Birds Eye**	0	0–10
Squash, cooked, frozen: ½ cup / **Seabrook Farms**	0	0–10
Squash, summer, in cheese sauce, frozen: 1 cup / **Green Giant** Boil-in-Bag	4	20–30
Squash, summer, sliced, frozen: 3.3. oz / **Birds Eye**	0	0–10
Stew, vegetable, canned: 7½ oz / **Dinty Moore**	8	40–50
Stew, vegetable, frozen: 3 oz / **Ore-Ida**	0	0–10
Succotash, canned: 1 cup / **Stokely-Van Camp**	1	0–10
Succotash, frozen: 3.3 oz / **Birds Eye**	1	0–10
Tomato paste, canned: 6 oz / **Contadina**	0	0–10
Tomato paste, canned: 6 oz / **Del Monte**	1	0–10
Tomato paste, canned: 3 oz / **Hunt's**	0	0–10
Tomato paste, canned: ⅔ cup / **Town House**	0	0–10

	FAT GRAMS	PERCENT OF CALORIES FROM FAT
Tomato puree, canned: 1 cup / **Contadina**	0	0–10
Tomatoes, canned: 1 cup unless noted		
Stewed / **Contadina**	0	0–10
Stewed / **Del Monte**	0	0–10
Stewed: 4 oz / **Hunt's**	0	0–10
Stewed / **Libby's**	0	0–10
Stewed / **Stokely-Van Camp**	0	0–10
Stewed / **Town House**	0	0–10
Wedges / **Del Monte**	0	0–10
Whole: ½ cup / **S and W Nutradiet**	0	0–10
Whole / **Stokely-Van Camp**	0	0–10
Whole / **Town House**	0	0–10
Whole, peeled / **Del Monte**	0	0–10
Whole, peeled: 4 oz / **Hunt's**	0	0–10
Whole, peeled / **Libby's**	0	0–10
Turnip greens, chopped, canned: 1 cup / **Stokely-Van Camp**	1	0–10
Turnip greens, chopped, frozen: 3.3 oz / **Birds Eye**	0	0–10
Turnip greens, chopped frozen: ½ cup / **Seabrook Farms**	0	0–10
Turnip greens, chopped w diced turnips, frozen: 3.3 oz / **Birds Eye**	0	0–10
Turnip greens, leaf, frozen: ½ cup / **Seabrook Farms**	0	0–10
Zucchini, frozen: 3.3 oz / **Birds Eye**	0	0–10
Zucchini, sticks, in light batter: 3 oz / **Mrs. Paul's**	9	40–50
Zucchini, in tomato sauce, canned: 1 cup / **Del Monte**	0	0–10

Vegetable Juices

Insignificant amounts of fat

Wines

No fat

Yeast

All kinds of yeast, including bakers and brewer's, have only trace amounts of fat.

Yogurt

1 cup unless noted 8 oz = ⅞ to 9/10 cup	FAT GRAMS	PERCENT OF CALORIES FROM FAT
All flavors: 8 oz container / **Dannon**	3	10–20
All flavors w fruit: 8 oz container / **Dannon**	2	0–10
All fruit flavors / **Lucerne** Lowfat	4	10–20
Apricot / **Sealtest Light n' Lively** Lowfat	2	0–10
Apricot / **Viva** Swiss Style Lowfat	2	0–10
Black cherry / **Sealtest Light n'** **Lively**	2	0–10
Black cherry / **Viva** Swiss Style Lowfat	2	0–10
Blackberry / **Viva** Swiss Style Lowfat	2	0–10
Blueberry **Europa** / 6 oz container	4	10–20

	FAT GRAMS	PERCENT OF CALORIES FROM FAT
Meadow Gold Western Sundae Style Lowfat	4	10–20
Sealtest Light n' Lively	2	0–10
Viva Swiss Style Lowfat	2	0–10
Blueberry-vanilla / **Sealtest Light n' Lively**	2	0–10
Boysenberry / **Meadow Gold** Western Sunday Style Lowfat	4	10–20
Boysenberry / **Viva** Swiss Style Lowfat	2	0–10
Cherry: 6 oz container / **Europa**	4	10–20
Fruit salad / **Viva** Swiss Style Lowfat	2	0–10
Lemon / **Sealtest Light n' Lively** Lowfat	2	0–10
Lemon / **Viva** Swiss Style Lowfat	2	0–10
Lemon-lime / **Sealtest Light n' Lively** Lowfat	2	0–10
Lemon-lime / **Viva** Swiss Style Lowfat	2	0–10
Orange, mandarin / **Meadow Gold** Western Sundae Style Lowfat	4	10–20
Orange, mandarin / **Sealtest Light n' Lively** Lowfat	2	0–10
Mandarin orange / **Viva** Swiss Style Lowfat	2	0–10
Peach		
Europa / 6 oz container	4	10–20
Meadow Gold Western Sundae Style Lowfat	4	10–20
Sealtest Light n' Lively Lowfat	2	0–10
Viva Swiss Style Lowfat	2	0–10
Peach melba / **Sealtest Light n' Lively** Lowfat	2	0–10
Pineapple / **Meadow Gold** Western Sundae Style Lowfat	4	10–20
Pineapple / **Sealtest Light n' Lively** Lowfat	2	0–10

	FAT GRAMS	PERCENT OF CALORIES FROM FAT
Pineapple coconut / **Viva** Swiss Style Lowfat	2	0–10
Pineapple-orange / **Viva** Swiss Style Lowfat	2	0–10
Plain: 8 oz container		
Made w whole milk	7	40–50
Lowfat (made w lowfat milk)	3.3	40–50
No fat (made w skim milk)	.4	0–10
Raspberry		
Europa / 6 oz container	4	10–20
Meadow Gold Western Sundae Style Lowfat	4	10–20
Sealtest Light n' Lively Lowfat	2	0–10
Viva Swiss Style Lowfat	2	0–10
Red cherry / **Viva** Swiss Style Lowfat	2	0–10
Strawberry: 6 oz container / **Europa**	4	10–20
Strawberry / **Meadow Gold** Western Sundae Style Lowfat	4	10–20
Strawberry / **Sealtest Light n' Lively** Lowfat	2	0–10
Strawberry / **Viva** Swiss Style Lowfat	2	0–10
Strawberry-banana / **Sealtest Light n' Lively** Lowfat	2	0–10
Strawberry fruit cup / **Sealtest Light n' Lively** Lowfat	2	0–10

FROZEN

	FAT GRAMS	PERCENT OF CALORIES FROM FAT
Danny Flip / 5 fl oz	1	0–10
Danny In-A-Cup / 8 fl oz	2	0–10
Danny Parfait / 4 fl oz	1	0–10
Danny Sampler / 3 fl oz	1	0–10
Danny-Yo / 3½ fl oz	1	0–10
Fruit: 8 fl oz / **Danny** In-A-Cup	2	0–10
Peach: ½ cup / **Sealtest**	1	0–10
Red raspberry: ½ cup / **Sealtest**	1	0–10

	FAT GRAMS	PERCENT OF CALORIES FROM FAT
Vanilla: ½ cup / **Sealtest**	1	0–10
Bars		
Carob-coated: 1 bar / **Danny** On-A-Stick	7.5	50–60
Chocolate-coated: 1 bar / **Danny** On-A-Stick	7.5	50–60
Uncoated: 1 bar / **Danny** On-A-Stick	1	10–20
Yosicle / 2½ fl oz	1	0–10

Fast Foods

ARBY'S

	FAT GRAMS	PERCENT OF CALORIES FROM FAT
Roast Beef Sandwich	15	30–40
Beef and Cheese Sandwich	22	40–50
Super Roast Beef Sandwich	28	40–50
Junior Roast Beef Sandwich	9	30–40
Swiss King Sandwich	34	40–50
Ham 'N Cheese Sandwich	17	30–40
Turkey Sandwich	19	40–50
Turkey Deluxe Sandwich	24	40–50
Club Sandwich	30	40–50

ARTHUR TREACHER'S

	FAT GRAMS	PERCENT OF CALORIES FROM FAT
Fish—two pieces	13	30–40
Chicken—two pieces	16	30–40
Shrimp—7 pieces	21	40–50
Chips	12	30–40
Krunch Pup	16	70–80
Cole Slaw	8	50–60
Lemon Luvs	16	50–60
Chowder	3	20–30
Fish Sandwich	15	20–30
Chicken Sandwich	12	20–30

BURGER CHEF

	FAT GRAMS	PERCENT OF CALORIES FROM FAT
Hamburger	13	40–50
Cheeseburger	17	50–60

	FAT GRAMS	PERCENT OF CALORIES FROM FAT
Double Cheeseburger	26	50–60
Big Shef	34	50–60
Super Shef	37	50–60
Skipper's Treat	37	50–60
French Fries	9	40–50
Shakes	11	20–30
Mariner Platter	24	30–40
Rancher Platter	38	50–60

BURGER KING

	FAT GRAMS	PERCENT OF CALORIES FROM FAT
Whopper	37	50–60
Double Beef Whopper	52	50–60
Whopper w Cheese	46	50–60
Double Beef Whopper w Cheese	61	50–60
Whopper Junior	20	40–50
Whopper Junior w Cheese	24	50–60
Whopper Jr. w Double Meat	29	50–60
Whopper Jr. Double Meat Pattie w Cheese	34	50–60
Hamburger	14	40–50
Hamburger w Cheese	18	40–50
Double Meat Hamburger	23	40–50
Double Meat Hamburger w Cheese	32	50–60
Steak Sandwich	21	30–40
Whaler	37	40–50
Whaler w Cheese	46	50–60
Onion Rings—Large	19	50–60
Onion Rings—Regular	13	50–60
French Fries—Large Bag	19	40–50
French Fries—Regular Bag	12	40–50
Chocolate Milkshake	11	20–30
Vanilla Milkshake	11	20–30
Apple Pie	12	40–50

CARL'S JR.

	FAT GRAMS	PERCENT OF CALORIES FROM FAT
Famous Star Hamburger	26	40–50
Super Star Hamburger	36	40–50
Old Time Star Hamburger	18	30–40
Happy Star Hamburger	11	30–40
Steak Sandwich	28	30–40
California Roast Beef Sandwich	10	20–30
Fish Fillet Sandwich	26	40–50
Original Hot Dog	19	40–50
Chili Dog	17	40–50
Chili Cheese Dog	20	40–50
American Cheese	3	60–70
11 oz Regular Salad w Condiments	3	10–20
2 oz Blue Cheese Dressing	19	80–90
2 oz Thousand Island Dressing	18	80–90
2 oz Lo-Cal Italian Dressing	0	0
French Fries	8	30–40
Onion Rings	18	50–60
Apple Turnover	15	40–50
Carrot Cake	18	40–50
20 oz Shake	7	10–20
20 oz Soft Drink	0	0

CHURCH'S FRIED CHICKEN

1 average piece, boned, dark	21	60–70
1 average piece, boned, white	23	60–70

DAIRY QUEEN / BRAZIER

Snacks and Desserts

Cone—Small	3	20–30
Cone—Regular	7	20–30
Cone—Large	10	20–30
Chocolate Dipped Cone—Small	7	40–50

	FAT GRAMS	PERCENT OF CALORIES FROM FAT
Chocolate Dipped Cone—Regular	13	40–50
Chocolate Dipped Cone—Large	20	40–50
Chocolate Sundae—Small	4	20–30
Chocolate Sundae—Regular	7	20–30
Chocolate Sundae—Large	9	20–30
Chocolate Malt—Small	11	20–30
Chocolate Malt—Regular	20	20–30
Chocolate Malt—Large	28	20–30
Float	8	20–30
Banana Split	15	20–30
Parfait	11	20–30
"Fiesta" Sundae	22	30–40
Freeze	13	20–30
"Mr. Misty" Freeze	12	20–30
"Mr. Misty" Float	8	10–20
"Dilly" Bar	15	50–60
"DQ" Sandwich	4	20–30
"Mr. Misty" Kiss	0	0

Fast Foods

	FAT GRAMS	PERCENT OF CALORIES FROM FAT
Hamburger	10	30–40
Cheeseburger	14	30–40
Big "Brazier"	23	40–50
Big "Brazier" w cheese	30	40–50
Big "Brazier" w Lettuce and Tomato	24	40–50
Super "Brazier" The "Half-Pounder"	48	50–60
Hot Dog	15	40–50
Hot Dog w chili	20	50–60
Hot Dog w cheese	19	50–60
Fish Sandwich	17	30–40
Fish Sandwich w cheese	21	40–50
French Fries	10	40–50
French Fries—Large	16	40–50
Onion Rings	17	50–60

HARDEE'S

	FAT GRAMS	PERCENT OF CALORIES FROM FAT
Hamburger	15	40–50
Cheeseburger	15	40–50
Huskie	41	50–60
Big Twin	26	50–60
French Fries—Small	13	40–50
French Fries—Large	21	40–50
Apple Turnover	14	40–50
Milkshake	10	20–30
Roast Beef Sandwich	16	30–40
Fish Sandwich	26	40–50
Hot Dog	22	50–60

KENTUCKY FRIED CHICKEN

Chicken Dinner:		
3 pieces chicken w mashed potatoes and gravy, cole slaw, and roll		
Original Recipe Dinner	46	40–50
Extra Crispy Dinner	54	50–60
Individual pieces, Original Recipe:		
Wing	10	50–60
Drumstick	8	50–60
Keel	13	40–50
Rib	14	50–60
Thigh	18	50–60

LONG JOHN SILVER'S SEAFOOD SHOPPES

Fish w Batter (2 piece order)	24	50–60
Fish w Batter (3 piece order)	36	50–60
Treasure Chest (1 piece fish & 3 peg legs)	29	50–60

	FAT GRAMS	PERCENT OF CALORIES FROM FAT
Chicken Planks (4 piece order)	23	40–50
Peg Legs w Batter (5 piece order)	33	50–60
Ocean Scallops (6 piece order)	12	40–50
Shrimp w Batter (6 piece avg order)	13	40–50
Breaded Oysters	19	30–40
Breaded Clams	25	40–50
S.O.S. Super Ocean Sandwich	30	40–50
Fryes	15	40–50
Cole Slaw	8	50–60
Corn on the Cob	4	20–30
Hush Puppies	7	40–50

MCDONALD'S

	FAT GRAMS	PERCENT OF CALORIES FROM FAT
Hamburger	10	30–40
Cheeseburger	13	30–40
Quarter Pounder	21	40–50
Quarter Pounder w Cheese	29	40–50
Big Mac	31	50–60
Filet-O-Fish	23	50–60
Egg McMuffin	20	50–60
Hot Cakes w Butter and Syrup	9	10–20
Scrambled Eggs	12	60–70
Pork Sausage	17	80–90
English Muffin (Buttered)	6	20–30
French Fries	11	40–50
Apple Pie	19	50–60
Cherry Pie	18	50–60
McDonaldland Cookies	11	30–40
Chocolate Shake	9	20–30
Vanilla Shake	8	20–30
Strawberry Shake	8	20–30

PIZZA HUT

	FAT GRAMS	PERCENT OF CALORIES FROM FAT

Serving size: one half of a 10-inch pizza (3 slices)

Thin 'N Crispy Pizza

	FAT GRAMS	PERCENT OF CALORIES FROM FAT
Beef	19	30–40
Pork	23	30–40
Cheese	15	20–30
Pepperoni	17	30–40
Supreme	21	30–40

Thick 'N Chewy Pizza

Beef	20	20–30
Pork	23	30–40
Cheese	14	20–30
Pepperoni	18	20–30
Supreme	22	30–40

STEAK N SHAKE

Steakburger	7	20–30
Steakburger w Cheese	13	30–40
Super Steakburger	12	20–30
Super Steakburger w Cheese	18	30–40
Triple Steakburger	17	30–40
Triple Steakburger w Cheese	30	40–50
Low Calorie Platter	14	40–50
Baked Ham Sandwich	22	40–50
Toasted Cheese Sandwich	13	40–50
Ham & Egg Sandwich	17	30–40
Egg Sandwich	10	30–40
Lettuce & Tomato	0.1	0–10
French Fries	10	40–50
Chili & Oyster Crackers (⅔ oz)	14	30–40
Chili Mac and 4 Saltines	12	30–40
Chili—3 Ways & 4 Saltines	16	30–40
Baked Beans	4	20–30

	FAT GRAMS	PERCENT OF CALORIES FROM FAT
Lettuce & Tomato Salad (1 oz, 1000 Island dressing)	15	70–80
Chef Salad	18	50–60
Cottage Cheese (½ cup)	4	30–40
Apple Danish	24	50–60
Strawberry Sundae	22	50–60
Hot Fudge Nut Sundae	34	50–60
Brownie Fudge Sundae	35	40–50
Apple Pie	18	30–40
Cherry Pie	14	30–40
Apple Pie a la Mode	25	40–50
Cherry Pie a la Mode	22	40–50
Cheese Cake	11	50–60
Cheese Cake w Strawberries	11	20–30
Brownie	12	40–50
Vanilla Ice Cream (1½ scoops)	12	50–60
Vanilla Shake	38	50–60
Strawberry Shake	40	50–60
Chocolate Shake	38	50–60
Orange Freeze	24	40–50
Lemon Freeze	25	40–50
Coca-Cola Float	17	20–30
Orange Float	17	20–30
Lemon Float	19	20–30
Root Beer Float	17	20–30
Orange Drink	0	0
Lemon Drink	0	0
Orange Juice	0.4	0–10
Coffee	0	0
Hot Tea	0	0
Iced Tea	0	0
Milk	8	40–50
Root Beer	0	0
Dr. Pepper	0	0
Hot Chocolate	19	20–30

TACO BELL

	FAT GRAMS	PERCENT OF CALORIES FROM FAT
Bean Burrito	12	30–40
Beef Burrito	21	40–50
Beefy Tostada	15	40–50
Bellbeefer	7	20–30
Bellbeefer w Cheese	12	30–40
Burrito Supreme	22	40–50
Combination Burrito	16	50–60
Enchirito	21	40–50
Pintos 'N Cheese	5	20–30
Taco	8	30–40
Tostada	6	30–40

WHITE CASTLE

French Fries	11	40–50
Cheeseburger	9	40–50
Hamburger	7	30–40
Fish (wo tartar sauce)	9	40–50

Index

Ale, 16
Almonds
  salted and flavored, 128
  unsalted and unflavored, 129–130
Angel food cake, 27–28
Appetizers, 1
Apples, 84
Arby's, 225
Arthur Treacher's, 225
Artichokes
  canned and frozen, 198
  fresh, 195
Asparagus
  canned and frozen, 198
  fresh, 195
Au jus gravy mix, 87
Avocados, 84

Baby food 3–15
  baked goods, 3
  junior, 10–15
    cereal, 10
    fruits and desserts, 11–12
    main dishes, 12–15
    vegetables, 15
  strained, 3–10
    cereal, 3–4
    fruits and desserts, 4–6
    juices, 7
    main dishes, 7–9
    vegetables, 10
Bacon, 109–110
  with baked beans, canned, 198
  with potatoes, canned, 211
  soups with, 175, 184
Baked beans 198–199
Baking chocolate 49–50
Baking powder, 15
Bamboo shoots, raw, 195
Banana pudding, 154
Barbecue sauce 169
Barley, pearled, 195
Bean soups, 175
Beans
  baked, 198–199
  canned and frozen 198–202
    black turtle, 199
    fava, 199
    green, 199–200
    kidney, 200
    lima, 201
    pinto, 201
    red, 201
    roman 201

Beans (*cont.*)
    salad, 201
    shellie, 201
    wax or yellow, 201–202
  fresh, 195–196
    great northern, 195
    lima, 195
    mung, 195
    pea beans, 196
    pinto, 196
    red, kidney, 196
    snap, 196
    white, 196
  in frozen dinners, 64
  refried, 119
Beechnuts, 130
Beef, 105–107
  bouillon, 176
  broth, 177
  corned, 110
  in dinner mixes, 68–69
  flavored rice, 160
  in frozen dinners, 64, 65, 66, 67
  gravy for, 87
  ground, 106
  meat entrees, canned, 115–116
  meat entrees, frozen, 116–118
  pot pies, 148
  soups, 175–177
Beef fat, 107
Beef stew
  canned, 115
  frozen, 118
  seasoning mix for, 172

Beets
  canned and frozen, 202
  fresh, 196
Beer, 16
Biscuits, 16
  buttermilk, 16
  refrigerator, 16
Black-eye peas, 209
Black olives, 133–134
Black turtle beans, 199
Blue cheese salad dressing, 165
Bologna, 110–111
Borscht, 176
Bouillon, 176–177
Brandies, 101
Brazil nuts, 130
Bread, 17–19
  rye, 18
  wheat, 18
  white, 19
Bread crumbs, 19
Bread mixes, 19–20
Breadsticks, 20
Breakfast bars, 135
Breakfast foods, frozen and prepared, 135–137
Broadbeans, 196
Broccoli
  fresh, 196
  frozen, 203
Broth, 177
Brown gravy, 87–88
Brown rice, 159
Brownies, 31
  mixes for, 58
Brussel sprouts, 203

Bundt cake, 28
Buns
  honey, 164
  sandwich, 161–162
Burger Chef, 225–226
Burger King, 226
Butter, 21
Butterbeans, 203
Buttermilk, 121
Butternuts, 130
Butters, 99
Butterscotch pudding, 154

Caesar salad dressing, 165
Cakes, 25–31
  frozen dessert, 25–27
  mixes, 27–30
  snack, 31–33
Candy, 33–35
  chocolate and chocolate
    covered bars, 33–34
  chocolate and chocolate
    bits, 34
  dietetic, 34–35
Carl's Jr., 227
Carrots
  canned and frozen, 204
  fresh, 196
Cashew nuts
  salted and flavored, 128
  unsalted and unflavored,
    130
Catsup, 52
Cauliflower
  fresh, 196
  frozen, 204

Celery, 196
  soup, cream of, 177
Cereals, 36–41
  for babies
    junior, 10
    strained, 3–4
  dry, 36
  to be cooked, 39–41
Cheddar cheese soup, 177
Cheese, 42–44
  cottage, 43–44
  foods, 44
  natural, 42–43
  pasteurized process, 43
  snacks, 47–48
  spreads, 44
Cheese snacks, 47–48
Cheese food, 44
Cheese sauce, 169
Cheese spreads, 44
Cheesecake, 25, 28
Chef style salad dressing,
  165–166
Chestnuts, 130
Chewing gum, 45
Chick peas
  canned, 204
  fresh, 196
Chicken
  bouillon, 176
  broth, 177
  canned, frozen and pro-
    cessed, 150–151
  flavored rice, 160
  fresh, 149
  in frozen dinners, 65, 67
  gravy for, 88–89

Chicken (cont.)
  pot pies, 148
  salad spread, 189
Chicken soup, 178–180
Chicken spreads, 189
Chili con carne, 119
Chiles, 119
  seasoning mix for, 172–173
Chinese foods, 45–47
  in frozen dinners, 65, 67
  mixed vegetables, 207
Chips, crisps and similar snacks, 47–49
Chocolate
  cakes, 25, 27, 29
  candy, 33–34
  chips, for baking, 49–50
  cookies, 54
  cupcakes, 26, 32
  dietetic candy, 34–35
  frosting, 82, 83
  ice cream 93–94, 95
  ice milk, 94
  pudding, 154–155
  toppings, 193
Chop suey, 45
  seasoning mix for, 173
Chowmein, 45–46
Chowder, 180–181
Church's Fried Chicken, 227
Clam chowder, 180
Clams, 75, 76
  canned and frozen, 75–76
  in frozen entrees, 79
Cocktail mixes, 50

Cocoa, 50–51
Coconut, 51
  pudding, 155
Coffee, 51
Coffee cake, 26, 31
Coleslaw dressing, 166
Collard greens
  fresh, 196
  frozen, 204
Condensed whole milk, sweetened, 121
Condiments, 52
Consommé, 181
Cookies, 53–57
  mixes and dough, 58–59
Corn
  canned and frozen, 204–206
  fresh, 196
Corn snacks, 48
Corned beef, 110
  spread, 189
Cornstarch, 60
Cottage cheese, 43–44
Cowpeas, 196
Crab, 75
  canned and frozen, 76
  in frozen entrees, 79
Crackers, 60–62
Cream, 62
Crepes, 135
Croutons, 20
Crumbcake, 26
Cucumber salad dressing, 166
Cucumbers, 196
Cupcakes, 26, 29, 31–32
Custard, 155

Dairy Queen, 227–228
Dandelion greens 196
Dessert mixes, 63
Deviled ham, 189
Diet bars, 63
Dietetic candy, 34–35
Dinner rolls, 162–163
Dinners, 64–70
    frozen, 64–68
    in mixes, 68–70
Donuts 32
    frozen, 137–138
Dried milk, 121
Duck, 149

Egg biscuits, 54
Egg rolls, 46
Eggplant, 96, 196
Eggs, 71–72
    fresh, 71–72
    fried, 71
    hard-boiled, 71
    imitation, 72
    omelet, 72
    scrambled, 72
Enchiladas
    in frozen dinners, 65, 120
    seasoning mix for, 173
English muffins, 124
Evaporated milk, 121

Farina, 39
Fast foods, 225–233
Fava beans, 199
Fig bars, 54
Filberts, 130

Flour, 80–81
Fish 73–75
    canned and frozen, 76
    fresh, 73–75
    in frozen dinners, 65, 66, 67, 68
    in frozen entrees, 79–80
Flavored milk beverages, 121–123
Flavorings, sweet, 80
Frankfurters, 111
    with baked beans, canned, 199
    buns, 161–162
    in frozen dinners, 64
    soup with, 175
    with spaghetti, canned, 188
French bread, 17
French dressing, 166
French fried potatoes, 197, 211–212
French toast, 135–136
Fried rice, seasoning mix for, 173
Fried rinds, 48
Fritters, 136
Frostings, 82–84
    packaged, 83–84
    ready to spread, 82–83
Frozen dessert, 93
Frozen yogurt, 223–224
Fruit, 84–85
    canned, frozen and dried, 85
    fresh, 84–85
Fruit juices, 85

Garbanzos. *See* Chick peas
Gelatin, 87
Goat milk, 121
Goose, 149–150
Grains, 82
Granola bars, 91
Grapefruit, 84
Gravies, 87–90
Great northern beans, 195
Green beans, 199–200
Green olives, 133–134
Green peas. *See* Peas, green
Grits, 40
Ground beef, 106
   seasoning mix for, 173

Ham
   with baked beans, canned, 199
   canned, whole, 112
   in frozen dinners, 66
   luncheon type, 112
   with potatoes, canned, 211
   soups with, 175
Ham spreads, 184–189
Hamburger
   buns, 161–162
   in dinner mixes, 68–70
   seasoning mix for, 172, 173
Hard rolls, 163
Hardee's, 229
Hash, 116
Hash brown potatoes, 212–213
Health foods, 91–92

Heart, 107
Herbs, 92
Hollandaise sauce, 169
Honey bread, 17
Hot dogs. *See* Frankfurters
Human milk, 121

Ice cream, 93–94
Ice cream bars, 95–96
Ice cream sandwich, 95
Ice milk, 94–95
Imitation eggs, 72
Italian bread, 17
Italian dressing, 167
Italian foods, 96–98. *See also specific food*
   in dinner mixes, 68
   in frozen dinners, 66, 67
   mixed vegetables, 206–208
   sauce for, 168–170
Italian sauce, 168–170

Jams, 99
Jellies, 99
Juice(s)
   fruit, 85
   strained for babies, 7
   vegetable, 217

Kale
   fresh, 196
   frozen, 206
Kentucky Fried Chicken, 229
Kidney beans
   baked, 198

canned and frozen, 200–201
fresh, 196
Kidneys, 107

Lamb, 108
Lard, 174
Lasagna, 96–97
Lentil soup, 181
Lentils, 196
Lettuce, 196
Lima beans
    canned and frozen, 201
    fresh, 195
Liqueurs, 101
Liver
    beef, 108
    calf, 108
    chicken, 149, 151
    hog, 108
    lamb 108
Liverwurst, 189
Lobster, 75
Long John Silver's Seafood Shoppes, 229–230
Lowfat milk, 121
Luncheon meat, 112–113

Macaroni, 103–104
    bag entrees, 103
    and beef, 103
    and cheese, 103–104
    in frozen dinners, 66
    and meatballs, 104
    plain, 103
McDonald's, 230

Malt liquor, 16
Manicotti, 97
Margarine, 21–22
    imitation, 22
Marmalade, 99
Matzo meal, 82
Matzos, 61
Mayonnaise, 104–105
    imitation, 105
Meal, 82
Meat, 105–115
    canned, cured, processed, 109–116
    fresh 105–109
    marinade, seasoning mix for, 173
Meat entrees
    canned, 115–116
    frozen, 116–118
Meat loaf
    in frozen dinners, 66
    frozen entrees, 117
    seasoning mix for, 173–174
Meat substitutes, 118–119
    vegetarian, 91–92
Meat balls
    in frozen dinners, 66, 67
    frozen entree, 117
    seasoning mix for, 173
    soup, 181
    with spaghetti, canned, 188
Mexican foods, 119–120
    in frozen dinners, 66–67
Milk 121
Minestrone soup, 181–182

Mint candy, 35
Minute rice, 159
Mixed nuts, 127–128
Mixed vegetables, canned and frozen, 206–208
Muffins, 123–125
Mung beans, 195
Mushroom gravy, 89
Mushroom soup, 182
Mushrooms
  canned and frozen, 208
  fresh, 196
Mustard, 52
Mustard greens
  fresh, 196
  frozen, 208

Natural cheese, 42–43
Navy beans. See Pea beans
Non-dairy creamers, 62
Noodles, 127–128
  chicken and, 151
  Chinese, 46–47
  in dinner mixes, 68, 69, 70
  in frozen dinners, 65, 67
  and noodle dishes 127–128
  in soups, 178–179, 186
Nuts
  salted and flavored, 128–129
  unflavored, unsalted, 129–131

Oatmeal, 40–41
  cookies, 56
Oils, 133

Okra
  fresh, 197
  frozen, 208
Olives, 133–134
Omelets, 72
Onion(s)
  bouillon, 176
  broth, 177
  canned and frozen, 208–209
  fresh, 197
Onion gravy, 89
Onion soup, 183
Oranges, 85
Ovaltine, 122
Oyster stew, 183

Pancakes
  frozen, 136
  mix, prepared, 136–137
Pasteurized process cheese, 43
Parsnips, 197
Pastrami, 113
Pastry, 137–138
  pie crust and pastry shells, 143
  pie filling, 143–144
  pie mixes, 142–143
  pie snacks, 144
  toaster, 138–139
Pastry shells, 143
Pea beans, 196
Pea soup, 183–184
Peanut butter, 189–190
Peanuts
  salted and flavored, 129

unsalted and unflavored, 130

Peas, green
    canned and frozen, 209–211
    fresh, 197

Pecans
    salted and flavored, 129
    unsalted and unflavored, 130–131

Pepperoni, 113

Peppers
    fresh, 197
    in Mexican food, 120
    stuffed, frozen, 206

Pickles, 139

Pie crusts, 143

Pie filling, 143–144

Pie mixes, 142–143

Pie snacks, 144

Pie-Tarts, frozen 138

Pies, 140–142

Pilaf, 160–161

Pinenuts, 131

Pinto beans
    canned, 201
    fresh, 196

Pistachio nuts
    pudding, 156
    salted and flavored, 129
    unsalted and unflavored, 131

Pizza, 145–147
    sauce for, 170

Pizza Hut, 231

Pizza rolls, 147

Plum pudding, 156

Popcorn, 147

Popovers, 163

Popsicles, 95

Pop-Tarts, 138–139

Pork, 108–109
    with baked beans, canned, 199
    in frozen dinners, 67
    gravy for, 89

Pot pies, 148

Pot roast, gravy for, 89

Potato(es)
    canned and frozen, 211–214
    fresh, 197
    sweet, 197

Potato snacks, 48

Potato soup, 184

Poultry. See also Chicken; Turkey
    canned, frozen and processed, 150–153
    flavored rice, 160
    fresh, 149

Pound cake, 27, 30

Preserves, 99

Pretzels, 153

Profile bread, 17

Pudding, 154–157

Pumpernickel bread, 17

Pumpkin, 214

Rabbit, 109

Radishes, 197

Raisin bread, 17

Ravioli, 97

Red beans, 201

Relishes, 139
Rhubarb, 85
Rice, 159–161
  brown, 159
  in dinner mixes, 69
  dishes, 160–161
  fast cooking, 159–160
  minute, 159
  pudding, 156
  in soups, 179, 185–186
  white, 159
Rice dishes, 160–161
Rolls
  dinner and soft, 161
  hard, 163
  sweet, 163–164
Roman beans, 201
Russian dressing, 167–168
Rutabagas, 197
Rye bread, 18
Rye flour 81

Salad beans, 201
Salad dressing, 165–169
Salami, 114
Salisbury steak
  in frozen dinners, 67
  meat entree, canned, 116
  meat entrees, frozen, 117–118
Saltines 61
Sandwich spreads, 190
Sauces, 52, 169–174
Sauerkraut, 214
Sausage, 114–115
Seafood, 73–80

fish, 73–75, 76–79
  frozen entrees, 79–80
  shellfish, 75, 75–76, 77, 78
Seasoning mixes 172–174
Sesame nut mix, 129
Shellfish, 75
  canned and frozen, 75–76, 77, 78
  fresh, 75
Shellie beans, 201
Sherbet, 95
Shortening, 174
Shrimp, 75
  canned and frozen, 78
  in frozen entrees, 79
  soup, cream of, 184
Skim milk, 121
Sloppy Joe
  canned, 116
  frozen, 118
  seasoning mix for, 174–175
Snack cakes, 31–33
Snack sticks, 48–49
Snacks
  cake, 31–33
  cheese, 47–48
  chips and crisps, 47–49
  corn, 48
  pie, 144
  snap beans, 196
  soda crackers, 61
Soft drinks, 174
Soup greens, in jar, 214
Soups, 175–188
Sour cream sauce, 170
Soy milk, 92

Soy sauce, 52
Soybean flour, 81
Soybeans, 197
Spaghetti
  dishes, 188–189
  in dinner mixes, 70
  in frozen dinners, 67
  plain cooked, 188
  sauce for, 170–171
  with sauce, frozen, 189
  with sauce, mixes, 189
Spam, 115, 190
Spanish rice, 161
  seasoning mix for 174
Spareribs, 109
Spices, 92
Spinach
  canned and frozen, 214–
    215
  fresh, 197
Spreads, 189–190
Squash
  fresh, 197
  frozen, 215
Steak, beef, 107
Steak N Shake, 231–232
Stew
  beef, 115, 118
  chicken, canned, 151
  meatball, 116
  Mulligan, 116
  oyster, 185
  vegetable, 215
Streusel cake, 30
Stroganoff sauce, 171
Stuffing mixes, 22–23

Succotash, 215
Sugar, 191
Sweet and sour sauce, 171
Sweet potato, 197
Sweet rolls, 163–164
Sweetbreads, 109
Sweeteners, 191

Taco(s)
  dinners, 120
  sauce, 52
  seasoning mix for, 174
  shells, 120
Taco Bell, 233
Tamales, 120
Tapioca, 156
Tartar sauce, 52
Tea, 193
Thousand island dressing,
  168
Toaster pastries, 138–139
Tomato paste, canned, 215
Tomato sauce, 171–172
Tomato soup, 185–186
Tomatoes
  canned, 215–216
  fresh, 197
Tongue, 109
Toppings, 193–194
Tortilla chips, 49
Tuna
  canned, 78–79
  in dinner mixes, 70
  fresh, 74
  in frozen entrees, 80

Tuna (*cont.*)
pot pies, 148
salad spread, 190
Turkey
canned, frozen and processed, 152–153
fresh, 150
in frozen dinners, 68
gravy for, 90
pot pies, 148
salad spread, 190
Turkey soup, 186
Turnip greens
canned and frozen, 216
fresh, 197
Turnips, 197
Turnovers, 138

Vanilla
cakes, 27
cookies, 57
frosting, 82–83, 84
ice cream, 94, 96
ice milk 95
Vanilla pudding, 156–157
Veal, 109
in frozen dinners, 68
parmagiana, frozen, 68
steaks, frozen, 115
Vegetable(s), 195–216
bouillon, 176–177
broth, 177
canned and frozen, 198–216
fresh, 195–197
Vegetable juices, 217

Vegetable shortening, 174
Vegetable soup, 186–188
Vegetable stew, 215
Vegetarian meat substitutes, 91–92
Vichyssoise, 188

Wafers, 57, 62
Waffles
frozen, 137
mix, prepared, 136–137
Walnuts, 131
Water chestnuts, 197
Watercress, 197
Wax beans, 201–202
Welsh rarebit, 44
Wheat bread, 18
Wheat flour, 81
White beans, 196
White bread, 19
White Castle, 233
White flour, 81
White sauce, 172
Whole milk, 121
Wine, 219
Worcestershire sauce, 52

Yeast, 221
Yellow beans, 201–202
Yogurt, 221–223
frozen, 223–224
salad dressing, 168–169

Ziti, baked, 98
Zucchini
canned and frozen, 216
fresh, 197

ABOUT THE AUTHOR

JEAN CARPER is a free-lance writer, specializing in consumer and health subjects. She has written numerous articles for national magazines (*Reader's Digest, Consumer Reports, Saturday Review, Today's Health*) in the medical field, including articles on food. She is the author of seven other books: *The All-In-One Calorie Counter; The All-In-One Carbohydrate Gram Counter; Stay Alive; Bitter Greetings: The Scandal of the Military Draft; The Dark Side of the Marketplace* (co-written with Senator Warren G. Magnuson); *Not With a Gun* and *Eating May be Hazardous to Your Health*. Ms. Carper writes a syndicated column for Princeton Features and is the national consumer reporter for Westinghouse Broadcasting. She is a graduate of Ohio Wesleyan University and lives in Washington, D.C.

How's Your Health?

Bantam publishes a line of informative books, written by top experts to help you toward a healthier and happier life.

☐	10350	**DR. ATKINS' SUPERENERGY DIET,** Robert Atkins, M.D.	$2.25
☐	13532	**FASTING: The Ultimate Diet,** Allan Cott, M.D.	$2.25
☐	13111	**THE COMPLETE SCARSDALE MEDICAL DIET,** Tarnower & Baker	$2.75
☐	13887	**A DICTIONARY OF SYMPTOMS,** J. Gomez	$2.75
☐	14221	**THE BRAND NAME NUTRITION COUNTER,** Jean Carper	$2.50
☐	13629	**SWEET AND DANGEROUS,** John Yudkin, M.D.	$2.50
☐	14209	**NUTRITION AGAINST DISEASE,** Roger J. Williams	$2.50
☐	12174	**NUTRITION AND YOUR MIND,** George Watson	$2.25
☐	13870	**HOW TO LIVE 365 DAYS A YEAR THE SALT FREE WAY** Brunswick, Love & Weinberg	$2.50
☐	12781	**THE PILL BOOK,** Simon & Silverman	$2.95
☐	13415	**WOMEN AND THE CRISIS IN SEX HORMONES,** The Seamans	$3.50
☐	12737	**THE ALL-IN-ONE CARBOHYDRATE GRAM COUNTER,** Jean Carper	$1.95
☐	12415	**WHICH VITAMINS DO YOU NEED?** Martin Ebon	$2.25
☐	13146	**FASTING AS A WAY OF LIFE,** Allan Cott, M.D.	$1.95
☐	13270	**THE ALL-IN-ONE CALORIE COUNTER,** Jean Carper	$2.25
☐	13259	**THE FAMILY GUIDE TO BETTER FOOD AND BETTER HEALTH,** Ron Deutsch	$2.50
☐	12023	**PSYCHODIETETICS,** Cheraskin, et al.	$2.25

Buy them at your local bookstore or use this handy coupon for ordering:

Bantam Books, Inc., Dept. HN, 414 East Golf Road, Des Plaines, Ill. 60016

Please send me the books I have checked above. I am enclosing $_____ (please add $1.00 to cover postage and handling). Send check or money order —no cash or C.O.D.'s please.

Mr/Mrs/Miss _____

Address _____

City_____State/Zip_____

HN—8/80

Please allow four to six weeks for delivery. This offer expires 12/80.

BE A WINNER
IN THE RACE FOR
FITNESS

These physical fitness titles give every member of the family the guidance they need for getting in shape and keeping fit. Choose the program most suited to you whether it be yoga, jogging, or an exercise routine. You'll feel better for it.

☐ 13418	**DR. SHEEHAN ON RUNNING**	$2.50
	George A. Sheehan	
☐ 12382	**GETTING STRONG** Kathryn Lance	$2.50
☐ 14158	**RUNNING FOR HEALTH AND BEAUTY**	$2.50
	Kathryn Lance	
☐ 11166	**JAZZERCISE** Missett & Meilach	$1.95
☐ 13061	**LILIAS, YOGA AND YOU** Lilias Folan	$2.25
☐ 13868	**AEROBICS** Kenneth H. Cooper	$2.50
☐ 13621	**AEROBICS FOR WOMEN** Cooper & Cooper	$2.50
☐ 13793	**THE AEROBICS WAY** Kenneth H. Cooper	$2.75
☐ 13617	**THE NEW AEROBICS** Kenneth H. Cooper	$2.50
☐ 13506	**CELLULITE** Nicole Ronsard	$2.50
☐ 11282	**THE ALEXANDER TECHNIQUE**	$1.95
	Sara Barker	
☐ 13379	**INTRODUCTION TO YOGA**	$2.25
	Richard Hittleman	
☐ 13847	**YOGA 28 DAY EXERCISE PLAN**	$2.25
	Richard Hittleman	

Buy them at your local bookstore or use this handy coupon for ordering:

Bantam Books, Inc., Dept. FI, 414 East Golf Road, Des Plaines, Ill. 60016
Please send me the books I have checked above. I am enclosing $_____ (please add $1.00 to cover postage and handling). Send check or money order —no cash or C.O.D.'s please.

Mr/Mrs/Miss _____

Address _____

City_____ State/Zip_____

FI—4/80

Please allow four to six weeks for delivery. This offer expires 10/80.

Bantam Book Catalog

Here's your up-to-the-minute listing of over 1,400 titles by your favorite authors.

This illustrated, large format catalog gives a description of each title. For your convenience, it is divided into categories in fiction and non-fiction—gothics, science fiction, westerns, mysteries, cookbooks, mysticism and occult, biographies, history, family living, health, psychology, art.

So don't delay—take advantage of this special opportunity to increase your reading pleasure.

Just send us your name and address and 50¢ (to help defray postage and handling costs).